What Makes Women Sick?

Brandeis Series on Jewish Women

The Hadassah International Research Institute on Jewish Women, established at Brandeis University in 1997 by Hadassah, the Women's Zionist Organization of America, Inc., supports interdisciplinary basic and applied research as well as cultural projects on Jewish women around the world. Under the auspices of the Institute, the Brandeis Series on Jewish Women publishes a wide range of books by and about Jewish women in diverse context and time periods.

Marjorie Agosín, *Uncertain Travelers: Conservations with Jewish Women Immigrants to America*, 1999

Rahel R. Wasserfall, *Women and Water: Menstruation in Jewish Life and Law*, 1999

Susan Sered, *What Makes Women Sick?: Maternity, Modesty, and Militarism in Israeli Society, 2000*

What Makes Women Sick?

Maternity, Modesty, and Militarism in Israeli Society

Susan Sered

Brandeis University Press

Published by University Press of New England

Hanover and London

Brandeis University Press

Published by University Press of New England, Hanover, NH 03755

Printed in the United States of America 5 4 3 2 1

Library of Congress Cataloging-in-Publication Data

Sered, Susan
What makes women sick? : maternity, modesty, and militarism in Israeli society / Susan Sered.
p. cm. — (Brandeis series on Jewish women)
Includes bibliographical references and index.
ISBN 1-58465-024-9 (cloth: alk. paper)—ISBN 1-58465-050-8 (pbk.: alk. paper)
1. Women—Health and hygiene—Social aspects—Israel. 2. Women—Israel—Social conditions. 3. Sex role—Israel. I. Title. II. Series.
RA564.85 .S47 2000
613'.04244'095694—dc21 00-022856

For my father, Robert M. Starr

Contents

Acknowledgments ix

INTRODUCTION: The Cultural Politics of Somatization 1

1. Collective Representations of Motherhood: The "Demographic Problem," Maternity Grants, and Abortion 22
2. The Reproductive Body: Pregnancy, Birth, Infertility, and Breastfeeding 41
3. The Militarized Body: Rape and the Woman Soldier 68
4. The Ritualized Body: Brides, Purity, and the Mikveh 104
5. The Scrutinized Body: Under the Knife, in Front of the Camera, and in Back of the Bus 122

CONCLUSION: Resisting Bodies 155

Notes 171

Works Cited 181

Index 191

Acknowledgments

I wish to thank the many Israeli women who have shared their anger, joy, and tears with me, talked politics with me, encouraged me as I developed into a mother and a scholar, and taught me and learned from me during the twenty years in which I have made my home in Israel.

This book was written in 1998–1999 while I was a Scholar-in-Residence at the Hadassah International Research Institute on Jewish Women at Brandeis University. I thank Brandeis Unversity and the HIRIJW for their support, and Bar Ilan University for providing me with the resources and time to sit quietly and write. I also thank Amy Avgar and the Israel Association for the Advancement of Women's Health for helping me track down data and for serving as an ongoing inspiration for this project.

I never would have been able to write this book without the support and encouragement of my husband, Yishai, who has helped me understand Israeli culture and Jewish sources. Much love and thanks to Yishai, Barak, Yoav, Asher, and Shifra for generously accompanying me to the United States where I found the distance I needed to appreciate what I had learned in Israel.

I would like to thank the Israel Women's Network for use of their excellent Information Center and archives. I wish to thank Misgav Ladach Hospital and especially Medical Director Dr. Michael Stark for allowing me to carry out field work on the maternity ward of the hospital. I thank all the new mothers at Misgav Ladach Hospital for their willingness to share their experiences with me. I thank the many women and attendants at mikvehs in Jerusalem who spent time talking to me about their own perspectives on Jewish law. I also thank my students at Bar Ilan University who have so eagerly talked to me about their experiences in the Israel Defense Forces.

This book has benefited from the generous and thoughtful help of three exceptional research assistants: Shirly Hering (the most dedicated young scholar I have ever met), Michelle Sternthal (a 1999 HIRIJW summer intern whose insights into anorexia helped me think through the connections between Jewish culture, illness, and the scrutiny of women's bodies), and Yvonne Deutsch. Special thanks to Leah Shakdiel, with hope that we will continue the dialogue sparked by working on this book. I thank Lynn Davidman for her astute comments and inspiring friendship. Orna Sasson-Levy graciously offered expert feedback on chapter 3; Rahel Wasserfall helped me avoid some dangerous conceptual pitfalls in chapter 4. Sharon Kaufman and Shulamit Reinharz helped me correct a multitude of errors and oversights, and offered me heartening and supportive feedback on the project. Ilsa Glazer's, Judith Lorber's, and Eyal Ben-Ari's readings of an earlier version of some of this material were essential in developing the theoretical thrust. I thank Deborah Greniman for her friendship and her insights into Jewish and Israeli culture. My appreciation to editor Phyllis Deutsch at University Press of New England for her encouragement and close reading of the manuscript.

S.S.

What Makes Women Sick?

Introduction

The Cultural Politics of Somatization

Israeli women are sicker and die younger then their counterparts in other western countries. Over the past decade the life expectancy of Israeli women has ranked in the vicinity of thirteenth to seventeenth in the world—trailing after Greece and Ireland, whereas the life expectancy of Israeli men has remained among the highest in the world—ranked second or third, following only Japan and Sweden (Israel Center for Disease Control 1997, 55–57). As is the case throughout Europe and North America, women in Israel outlive men, yet Israeli women's survival advantage is only *half* that of the average for European women.[1]

My own awareness of the poor health profile of Israeli women began in the mid-1980's when I carried out research among elderly Jewish women who had come to Israel from Kurdistan and other parts of Asia and North Africa in the first decades of the twentieth century (Sered 1992). Despite my efforts to encourage the women to talk to me about their religious beliefs and customs, their conversations almost always had to do with illness—with how Sima's legs hurt and how Rachel's pregnant daughter is bleeding and that Sarah's granddaughter seems to be starving herself and which doctor at the neighborhood clinic said what and the *zaddik* (holy man) in Petach Tikvah who cured Shlomo's weak heart and the herbs Mazal bought at the *shuk* (outdoor market) that clean out the blood in the early spring and the upcoming trip to a tomb of a saint who specializes in fertility problems and the blood tests Zehava has been sent to take and how old age brings with it aches and pains. It has taken me twenty years and a stint of field work in Okinawa (where women are rarely ill and even more rarely talk about being ill), to understand the extent to which illness is a constitutive part of the cultural and corporeal experiences of Israeli women.

This book represents my efforts—as a feminist and as an anthropologist—to expose and explicate some of the cultural practices that directly and indirectly make Israeli women sick. The focus of this book lies at the juncture of cultural constructions of femaleness and cultural constructions of illness in Israeli society. I hope to show that these two constructions take place in tandem; that femaleness is constructed via reference to illness and that constructions of illness incorporate notions of femaleness. The linchpins of this analogy include cultural understandings of femaleness and illness as states that need supervision and treatment, and cultural understandings of maleness and health as normative states that are superior to—and hold legitimate authority over—femaleness and illness.

The dialectical model that I develop in this book treats illness in Israeli women *both* as a product and byproduct of unjust gender practices and ideologies *and* as an intrinsic part of the Israeli gendering program itself. Gender hierarchy (in various forms, which I spell out throughout this volume) makes women ill, which generates and reinforces beliefs in female corporeal inferiority, which justifies the subordination of women (after all, women are weak and inferior creatures), which makes women ill. Bolstered by a cultural consensus that treats health, illness, and gender as manifestations of biological "truths," this cycle has proven very hard to break.

Gender and Illness in Israel: An Overview of the Evidence

Gendered patterns of sickness start young: Among sixth and seventh grade pupils 30.6% of boys and 41.3% of girls report suffering from dizziness, or headaches, stomachaches or backaches more than once a week; by tenth and eleventh grade the percentage of boys with these symptoms drops to 29.1% while the percentage of girls increases to 48.1%—close to half of all girls (Harel, Kaneh and Rahav 1997, 219). Throughout adulthood Israeli women report a higher rate than Israeli men of many of the most common and debilitating chronic diseases: diabetes, heart disease, kidney disease, ulcer, asthma, and hypertension (Israel Central Bureau of Statistics, cited in Avorva et al. 1996). Of the one thousand women who returned a health questionnaire published in the popular Israeli women's magazine *At*, one in three women had suffered at least one miscarriage; one in four had at least one abortion; the average number of pregnancies was 3.4; and almost one in eight of the married women had undergone some kind of fertility treatment. Fully three quarters of the women reported that they suffer from headaches; one third reported suffering from backaches; more than one quarter from chronic fatigue; and one quarter of the women reported using some kind of painkiller on a regular basis (Avgar and Gordon 1997).[2]

In another survey, Hana Eshed (1991) found that close to 40% of Israeli women between the ages of twenty and sixty reported feeling stress, anxiety, or depression. As Israelis age, the health disparity between men and women increases: A study of seventy-year-olds in Jerusalem revealed that more women than men suffer from cardiovascular disease, respiratory problems, chronic fatigue and mental disorders, and more than twice as many women as men were afflicted with joint and muscular conditions (such as arthritis) that result in chronic pain and disability. Perhaps not surprisingly, elderly women are more likely than elderly men to be living alone and subsisting solely on social security benefits (cited in Ifrah 1999, 130).[3]

Compared to women in the fifteen European Community countries that participated in a large-scale 1995 study, Israeli women had the third highest rates of mortality resulting from ischemic heart disease; Israeli men ranked significantly better—ninth (cited in Ifrah 1999, 97–99). Israeli women's mortality and morbidity rates from cancer are also comparatively high, while Israeli men's mortality and morbidity rates from cancer are comparatively low (Hoffman and Avgar 1998). In an analysis of forty European and North American countries in 1990, Israeli women ranked tenth highest in all-site incidence of cancer, in contrast to Israeli men who ranked thirty-third (cited in Ifrah 1999, 55).

Discrepancies between the comparatively good health of Israeli men and the comparatively bad health of Israeli women suggest that whatever is making women sick transcends the health care delivery system. And, in fact, medical care in Israel is readily available, affordable, regulated and subsidized by the government, on a technological level commensurate with the most developed Western countries, and for the most part operated on a not-for-profit basis. The doctor–patient ratio is very high (one doctor for every 217 individuals), and medical professionals are trained to standards equal to those of other developed countries (Hoffman and Avgar 1998). Israeli women make extensive use of the medical system: Women visit family doctors 20% more often and medical specialists 60% more often than men and hospitalization rates for women are 33% higher than for men (Reiss 1998, 79ff). Since the earliest years of the state, the government has provided virtually free prenatal care and obstetrical care, services that one would expect to see associated with good health outcomes for women. Yet, the services have not succeeded in keeping Israeli women as healthy as their counterparts in other countries with comparably good health care systems.

Blame for the poor health status of Israeli women does not appear to lie either with the medical system (at least not in a directly measurable way) or with "faulty" Jewish genes. In a study suggesting that environmental or cultural factors rather than genetic ones are to blame, Bryna Shatenstein and Jeremy Kark (1995) found that the cumulative mortality rates for Jewish women living in Israel are significantly higher than the rates for Jewish women living in Montreal (the one North American population for which reliable comparative statistics are available). And, according to Anneke Ifrah, "Studies have indicated that among certain [ethnic] origin groups, there is a significant increase in risk [of breast cancer] with increasing duration of residence in Israel, particularly among North African immigrants, whose risk increased by 75% after thirty years [in Israel]" (1999, 63–64).

Constructing Gender and Constructing Illness

Neither health/illness nor gender is a biological given: Cultures construe a variety of conditions as constituting illness or health,[4] just as cultures construe a variety of traits as characterizing masculinity or femininity. Gender and health/illness tend to be especially compelling cultural constructs because of their respective biological credentials or points of reference. In both instances, the body is borrowed to lend an aura of realness and certainty to cultural formulations (Scarry 1985, 12; Bolin 1992, 79).[5] In Israeli culture, for example, the biological presence of wombs confirms beliefs that women rather than men are the appropriate and "natural" caretakers of children (and by extension, of the handicapped, infirm, wounded, and elderly).

There are important correspondences between the workings of gender construction and the workings of health/illness construction. In each of these cases certain kinds of corporeality are created both through actions that mold or mark the body (for example, diet) and through conceptualizations of the body that attribute significance to particular corporeal markers (such as musculature). Put differently, gender and health/illness are conceptually constructed and physically imprinted onto human bodies in such a way that members of a culture (including the healthy/sick or gendered person him/herself) perceive them to be natural or objective conditions and logical conceptual schema for organizing society. What distinguishes Jewish Israeli society are the particular ways in which the cultural construction of health/illness and the cultural construction of gender interpenetrate. That interpenetration, the twicefold "borrowing" of the body to lend credence to conceptual formulations, results in some very persuasive cultural patterns.

Ideologies of gender difference framed in dichotomous and corporeal terms are deeply rooted in Jewish culture. The Biblical creation story, known by every Israeli schoolchild, tells that the first man and first woman were formed out of different physical substances: man out of earth and woman out of bone, and that women's destiny is to experience suffering pursuant to her female physiology. Noncorporeal identity, in contrast, is presented in gender-neutral terms in an adjacent Biblical narrative in which both men and women are created in God's image (Genesis 1:27, and 2:7, and 2:22). This literary juxtaposition can be understood as sacralizing a gender schema in which difference is conceptualized primarily in terms of physiology rather than in terms of moral virtues or mental abilities, a pattern that continues to this day to characterize Jewish Israeli culture. Gender differences reified through reference to immutable biological characteristics and reference to divine decree—the alliance of the "natural" and the "supernatural" in the cultivation of gender—make for very potent cultural material.

Israeli history has added some new spins to traditional Jewish gender schemas. The Zionist image of the *sabra*[6] was a radical reconstruction of the "effeminate" and pious scholar of the European Jewish ghettos. In Israeli Zionist cultural history the creation of the "new Jew" or "muscle Jew"—the quintessentially masculine farmer and warrior—was meant to replace the pale, weak, intellectual, sensitive, and victimized Jew of the shtetl (Boyarin 1997). Unfortunately, this reconstruction offered little to women: The early kibbutzim pushed women out of productive agricultural work as quickly as the pre-state military organizations and then the Israel Defense Forces (IDF) pushed women out of combat roles. The ideal Zionist was healthy, strong, and male: a farmer and a warrior. Not farmers but rather consumers and service providers, not warriors but rather those in need of protection, Israeli women have inherited a gendered corporeal culture in which "not healthy" and "not strong" are construed as feminine traits.

This highly gendered cultural formulation plays out in some very dramatic ways in the life experiences of Israeli women. As members of the "weaker" sex, women are thought to be vulnerable to rape at the hands of the enemy. This understandably gripping collective fear underpins the exclusion of women from combat positions in the IDF. One corollary of the exclusion of women from combat is that women soldiers are neither armed nor adequately trained in self-defense; without arms or self-defense skills, women soldiers are vulnerable to sexual harassment and violence. Incidents of sexual harassment and violence, in turn, make women ill (Koss 1994) and reinforce cultural conceptualizations of women as essentially weak and vulnerable. A second corollary of the exclusion of women from combat is that women are thought to lack the military experience and understanding necessary to set state policy. Outside of the loop of military decision-making institutions, women as a group have little say regarding the continued militarization of Israeli society, and continue to find their bodies enlisted in—conscripted into—a national culture in which being female and being weak/ill/vulnerable (or being male and being healthy/strong/assertive) mutually co-define.

The cross-fertilization of cultural formulations of femininity and weakness/illness/vulnerability is reified by law and custom. Israel was one of the first countries in the world to pass legislation on behalf of women workers. The Women's Labor Law of 1954 stipulates that "The Ministry of Labor is authorized, by regulation, to prohibit or limit the employment of women at any work, at any production process or at any place of work which is liable to particularly harm the health of a woman worker." Yet as Natalie Rein points out, this legislation was aimed at protecting women's bodies, not their rights (1980, 52 ff.). Knesset (Parliament) member Esther Vilenska (of Maki, Israeli Communist Party) insightfully argued during the August 2, 1954, Knesset debate prior to passing the law, that the proposed legislation related solely to prohibiting night work (which was believed to be dangerous for women and liable to take a toll on their health) and to maternity leave (which was seen as a matter of national demographic importance). The proposed legislation completely disregarded issues such as wage discrimination and discriminatory hiring, firing, and promotion practices. In this influential bit of "protective" legislation, women were depicted as inherently vulnerable to ill health, and employers were discouraged from hiring women because of restrictions on the conditions of their employment. At the same time, Israel's protective legislation (like similar legislation in other countries) has not kept women out of some of the most dangerous professions (hospital nursing with exposure to radiation, toxic chemicals, and germs) or even out of professions specifically dangerous to pregnant women (teachers, for example, are likely to be exposed to German measles [Scott 1984]), but has contributed to keeping women in "pink collar" jobs at salaries low enough to virtually guarantee economic vulnerability and the feminization of poverty with its attendant health risks.

Dominating Institutions: Competition and Collusion

Cross-culturally, different institutions wax and wane as major players in the work of gendering. These institutions sometimes compete and sometimes collude. The institutions most salient to gendering in contemporary Israel include the state, the religious establishment, the media, the consumer economy, and the medical establishment. Each of these institutions rests on somewhat (not totally) distinct ideological bases, historical foundations, and organizational structures. Israeli women are drawn into not one but several patriarchal narratives that merge to form a patriarchal "bricolage" or "mosaic" that is different from those at work in other Western or even other Middle Eastern societies. The salience and power of the various institutional narratives shift over time, a process that tends to elicit a great deal of attention and commentary in Israel's highly literate, self-aware, media-driven society.

Each gendering institution has it own vision of and agenda for women's bodies. For the religious establishment, the purity and modesty of women's bodies is of paramount importance; the state needs fertile women's bodies to bear and raise the next generation of citizens; the consumer economy frames women as physically attractive and as insatiable shoppers; and the medical establishment understands women's bodies to be especially prone to disease and in need of expert management. It should not be surprising that these competing agendas lead to inter-institutional conflict and to sickeningly contradictory demands being made upon women's bodies. Orthodox religious demands for a "pure" female body, national demands for maternal female fecundity, and capitalist demands for a sexualized and thin female consumer converge to draw women into a corporeal culture in which women's bodies are doomed to failure and sentenced to lifelong supervision and treatment at the hands of the medical establishment. As I show in chapter 5, women's bodies repeatedly become bargaining chips, booty, or the battlefield upon which political machinations and conflicts are enacted.

The state, with its power to unify and enforce bodily practices, is probably the most important player in the construction of female corporeality in Israel. Israeli women, like Israeli men, spend formative early adult years in the total institutional setting of the IDF, where their bodies are molded in very particular ways. In patriarchal cultures, according to Nira Yuval-Davis, men defend the symbolic construct known as "womenandchildren." She explains, "[G]endered bodies and sexuality play pivotal roles as territories, markers and reproducers of the narratives of nations and other collectivities . . . [G]ender relations are at the heart of cultural constructions of social identities and collectivities as well as in most cultural conflicts and contestations" (1997, 39). We shall see in chapter 3 that in Israeli discourse women's bodies are often framed as "the body" that is defended. This framing gives legitimacy to controlling women's bodies—otherwise the whole military effort is meaningless. Simultaneously, it draws women into the national project through constructing a discourse of the vulnerability of "womenandchildren" to attack, and especially to rape, at the hands of the enemy. In the defense of "womenandchildren," even the healthiest and strongest women become assimilated into the category of the weak, sick, and infirm—a category that itself is feminized through cultural associations linking male gender to health and female gender to illness.

The gendering agendas of the state and of the religious establishment are considerably different, yet they are not independent of one another. Contemporary Israeli society comprises a complex mixture of secular and religious institutions (Sobel and Beit-Hallahmi 1991). Although in most ways Israel resembles other Western democracies, Orthodox Judaism in Israel is institutionalized through a system of state-run religious schools, state-funded synagogues and religious services, municipal religious councils, Orthodox rabbinical control of weddings and divorces, and municipal and national chief rabbis whose public stature and Jewish legal rulings carry a great deal of cultural weight. Shlomit Levy, Hanna Levinsohn, and Elihu Katz (1993) found that 14% of Jewish Israelis consider themselves to be strictly observant of Jewish law, 24% observant to a great extent, 41% somewhat observant, and only 21% not observant at all. The vast majority of Israelis continue to practice at least some traditional Jewish rituals, and study after study reports that most Israelis believe in God and embrace at least some elements of Jewish doctrine (Kedem 1991).[7] Seen by many as the representatives of the "authentic" Jewish heritage, Orthodox rabbis hold a kind of iconic or mythic power in Israeli culture. While Orthodox political parties have never constituted more than a minority voice, they have always had representatives in the Knesset, and have been part of almost all government coalitions since the founding of the state.

I am particularly interested in cases in which institutions with divergent goals and values collude in the control of women. For example, the state (through legislation), rabbis (through sermons and pamphlets), and doctors (through participation in the system of hospital committees that grant or deny women abortions) all cooperate in limiting abortion and encouraging fertility. Similarly, the state gives monetary childbirth grants to women, charismatic rabbis give fertility blessings, and the advertising industry sells women myriad pieces of infant equipment (and sells all kinds of other products through the use of "cute" babies in commercials). As I shall argue throughout this book, several powerful institutions, each with its own distinct ideological and organizational structure, encourage women in the national mission of motherhood, address attention to women's bodies, and construe women's bodies as needing institutional help and guidance. Surprisingly often, women experience these various institutions as indistinguishable; sometimes the institutions even act as agents or function as veils for one another.

Jewish Israeli women's bodies are culturally understood to be unpredictable and unreliable—in need of investigation and mending. Perhaps women are in particular need of surveillance because of deep, usually unvoiced fears that women may not be fully invested in the patriarchal system (although the system is dependent upon women's labors). These fears are given voice when women who protest military actions are accused of caring more for the safety of their own sons than for the good of the state collective (see Conclusion), when women who insist on natural childbirth or exclusive breastfeeding are accused of caring more for themselves than for their babies (see chapter 2), and when women who dress in ways that please their own sensibilities are accused of polluting the morals of the community (see chapter 5). Suspicions of women's potential treachery (often glossed as "weakness") bolster the conviction that women must be watched and controlled, and translate into cultural patterns of keeping women under surveillance and dependent upon patriarchal institutions to protect and heal them.

Circumcision brings Jewish men into the covenant community once and for all. Even the most secular Israeli parents circumcise their boys so that they won't look different from other boys. Women's status in the covenant community is more precarious, in need of negotiation and testing, endlessly scrutinized through, for example, monthly rituals at the *mikveh* (ritual bath; see chapter 4). What women do with their bodies, or what is done to women's bodies, can endanger not only women but the entire collective. Israeli brides are told that failure to properly observe the laws of menstrual purity and ritual immersion can endanger their husbands, children, and all of the IDF soldiers fighting for national security. These sorts of ideologies situate women on the margins of the covenant community; women's membership in the community is neither permanent nor absolute (which is perhaps what lies behind the national fear of women's fighting on the front lines where they could be captured by enemy soldiers; see chapter 3).

In Israeli culture men's bodies are treated as quantifiable. Each soldier is assigned a health profile score by the IDF—a number that, particularly for male soldiers, is understood to summarize their corporeal assets—signifying for men fitness, or lack of fitness, for combat duty (IDF profiles are notoriously difficult to change). Male deaths are quantified in body counts and in military decisions regarding how many soldiers or policemen to send to each trouble spot. Football players have numbers; representatives in political parties are ranked by number; even the Bible counts men over the age of twenty, but not women (the counting, significantly enough, is for military purposes; Numbers 1:3). While men's infertility is numbered and knowable (expressed in terms of sperm count and motility), women's bodies are endlessly explored to discover the mysterious roots of infertility. Women's bodies are not quantifiable but rather complex—the object of "thick" (qualitative) analysis. Unquantifiable means unknowable and potentially uncontrollable, leading to ceaseless effort to "plumb" the mysteries of women's bodies in order to control (know) them.

In the quest to know, control, and cultivate Israeli women's bodies, the medical establishment plays the most visible role. Kathryn Pauly Morgan (1998) characterizes medicalization as the expansion of the medical jurisdiction so that individuals, groups, and institutions increasingly view issues, conditions, or situations in medical terms. Medicalization works through macro and micro processes; interlocking institutions allow medical conceptualizers to attain and preserve their status as possessors of authoritative knowledge. In Israel, as in many other Western societies, women are singled out as targets for medicalization. Where Israel may differ from other Western countries is in the extent of medicalization: Women's bodies (or more precisely, women's wombs) are understood to be a national resource, and women are conscripted into a highly efficient and well-developed medical system to a degree that surpasses the experiences of women elsewhere.

We shall see throughout this book that in Israeli society the attitudes of medicalization—especially regarding women's bodies—are shared not only by doctors but also by teachers, government officials, politicians, the IDF, the media, rabbis, mikveh attendants, and family members, all of whom "look out" for female illness. I shall describe situations in which a variety of institutions collude in the project of framing women as ill, and then tacitly (and sometimes explicitly, through legislation; see chapter 1) agree to allow the medical institution to "care" for women's bodies.

I find it significant that the parts of women's bodies that are particularly singled out for medical attention tend to be those parts that are understood as signifiers of female gender: wombs and breasts. In chapter 1 we will look at the medicalization of abortion. As we shall see in chapter 2, the cultural construction of high rates of infertility in Israel leads large numbers of women to submit their bodies to medical testing and treatment. In chapter 5 we will look at recent advertisements in the Israeli media for breast augmentation and reduction surgery—an obvious case of culture enlisting women's organs into the medical project, this time for reasons of fashion (often construed in terms of sexual attractiveness) rather than maternity. A fundamental component of medicalization is that once a person is viewed as a patient, he or she comes into legitimate range for ongoing medical surveillance. We shall see in chapter 5 that scrutiny of women's bodies, and debates over who has the right to scrutinize women's bodies, are reiterated themes in Israeli culture.

For women, the bottom line of medicalization is the wholesale conversion of normal bodily structures and processes to pathology. This conversion means that women turn to physicians more than men do (reflected in the higher rates of physician visits, hospitalization, and so on), and that women assimilate a concept of their bodies that is unhealthy. Concern with health and illness permeates women's discourse. Both in my fieldwork and in my own daily life in Israel I repeatedly hear women (far more than men) sigh and exclaim, "The most important thing [*ha-ikar*] is health, only health" and punctuate conversations with the words "He [or she or you] should be healthy." In contemporary Israeli culture, if you are a woman you are likely to seek medical attention for being "too" thin (maybe you are anorectic) or for being "too" fat (maybe you need a diet). Israel has an unusually high percentage of girls who at age eleven are already dieting, although there is no evidence that Israeli girls are especially overweight (Harel, Kaneh, and Rahav 1997). Fertility demands medical supervision, and so does infertility. Menstruation elicits medical attention (premenstrual syndrome, cramps, "heavy" bleeding), attention that may be augmented by the mikveh establishment sending women for medical help in "regulating" their periods so that their ovulation will fit the timing of sexual intercourse demanded by the laws of *niddah* (menstrual impurity; see chapter 4). And menopause is medicalized, requiring hormone replacement therapy to ward off osteoporosis and hot flashes.

"Syndromes" such as PMS and menopause are manifestations of cultural conceptualizations of women being sick by nature and in need of medical treatment (Morgan 1998, 103). In Israel, women's bodies often are described as "special" or as having "unique needs," conceptualizations that fuel beliefs in women's inherent weakness and inability to contribute actively to national defense. This conceptualization was at work in the discussion of protective legislation for women that I presented earlier. In the 1990s, "women's health centers" run by the seminationalized health insurance organizations *kupot holim* (sick funds) have sprung up throughout Israel. It may feel uncomfortable to criticize these centers since they provide screening for breast and cervical cancer and for osteoporosis, but the absence of comparable "men's health centers" does imply that women are "uniquely" sick and that their sickness is located in their most "female" organs.

Paradoxically, the intense medicalization of women's bodies does not necessarily mean that women receive better health care. Studies both in Israel and the United States show that women who seek help for chest pain are often told that the pain is psychosomatic or simple indigestion, and sent home. As a result, Israeli women fare worse than men during and after acute myocardial infarctions and bypass surgery. When they are actually admitted for surgery they are sicker, slower to recover, and more likely to die both during hospitalization and in the year following discharge (Swirski, Kanaaneh, and Avgar 1998, 13).[8] Nor does intense medicalization guarantee good health. In a self-perpetuating cycle, extensive use of medication and exposure to medical procedures may actually create a body that is sick and weak.

The Somatic Consequences of Oppression

Two decades ago, in her pioneering analysis of women in Israeli culture, Leslie Hazleton (1977) drew attention to the discrepancies between what is promised women (both by law and by the Zionist myth of equality) and what they actually can attain. The rhetoric of equality and shared purpose in building the Jewish state that Israeli women are raised on is poor preparation for the reality of second-class salaries and exclusion from leadership roles that has persisted from the first years of the state through the present time.

A fascinating longitudinal study carried out by Lotte Salzberger suggests that Israeli women more than Israeli men manifest their experiences of oppression through somatic symptoms. Among 360 married Israeli couples in families classified as moderately or severely economically disadvantaged, functional impairment due to illness increased over a ten-year period by 350% for women and by just 58% for men. Women were more likely than men to report multiple health problems, which they attributed to pregnancy, childbirth, persistent side effects of previous illness, and family stress. Pushing Salzberger's findings a bit further, it could be that women are more likely than men to suffer from multiple sources of deprivation and powerlessness both inside and outside the home, a situation that leads to especially poor health. Alternatively, it may be the case that in Israeli families, as in Israeli society in general, women physically bear and symbolically embody the distress of the collective.

A growing corpus of evidence illustrates how women's subordinate status in a variety of cultures is exhibited in illness-causing social practices such as overwork, lesser access to food, complications of frequent childbearing and sexually transmitted diseases, and infections and hemorrhages following genital mutilation or other dismembering operations (Lorber 1997, 14–15). Conversely, access to roles of social prestige and economic significance seem to have beneficial effects on women's health.[9] The question of gender hierarchy and life expectancy has been explored in an analysis of conjugal power in Tokugawa, Japan. Following the life courses of 360 couples in one village, G. William Skinner found that among equally matched spouses (identified by relatively late marriage for women and a small gap in spousal ages) women were long-lived vis-à-vis their husbands. Having married at a more mature age, these women would have been emotionally and practically well equipped to stand up to husband and mother-in-law. Among what he calls "high husband power" couples, women's life expectancy decreased vis-à-vis men's. These women not only married younger, but the gap in age between the husband and wife was larger, leading, Skinner argues, to a more hierarchical relationship.

Among couples in which the age difference was very great and the husband predeceased the wife by many years, the widow's life expectancy tended to be quite long, indicating that the freedom of widowhood may have increased life expectancy for women. Skinner concludes that, "Unrelieved powerlessness and structural vulnerability to oppression—and, we must assume, to the consequent overwork and physical hardship—are in the long run life-negating. The data . . . on conjugal power . . . [demonstrate] that the experience of wielding effective power within the family is life-enhancing" (1993, 259).

Perhaps the most striking piece of evidence linking women's status to life expectancy comes from Okinawa (Japan). Okinawa is the only society in the contemporary world in which women are the official, acknowledged leaders of the mainstream religion (see Sered 1999). Priestesses embody holiness and divinity, receive food and money offerings from the community, and carry out rituals that are understood to safeguard the health and well-being of all members of society. While the high status of women is most obvious in regard to religious matters, women generally encounter little discrimination, there are no popular beliefs about the inferiority of women's bodies or souls, and women are respected for their work as farmers, merchants, and mothers. Perhaps not surprisingly, Okinawan women have the longest life expectancy of women anywhere in the world today. I draw particular attention to the large survival advantage Okinawan women have vis-à-vis Okinawan men, a situation that is the very reverse of the Israeli one.

LIFE EXPECTANCY

Okinawa Prefecture (1990): 76.67 years (men), 84.47 years (women) **+7.8 years difference**

Japan (1990): 76.04 years (men), 82.07 years (women) **+6.03 years difference**

Israel (1990–1994): 75.1 years (men), 78.8 years (women) **+3.7 years difference**

(Okinawa Prefectural Office 1994; Israel Central Bureau of Statistics 1998).

Responsibility without Authority

What I loosely call "oppression" or "subordination"—systematic exclusion from positions of prestige and power, inferior access to valued resources, and cultural valuation as lesser or inferior—takes shape in different cultures in various "sickening" ways, some of which I shall discuss in detail later on in this book. At this point I would like to draw attention to one particular manifestation of oppression that seems to me to be especially characteristic of Israeli culture: the pattern of attributing collective responsibility to women and collective authority to men.[10] Women are encouraged to believe that their bodies carry weighty public and communal significance—that their wombs bear the responsibility to replace the six million Jews who died in the Holocaust and to produce the next generation of soldiers and citizens of the Jewish state. Yet all of the significant decision-making entities in Israel are absolutely dominated by men. Women are responsible for bearing and raising children, yet lack the authority to determine if their children will live or die. The corporeal ramifications of this pattern are far-reaching.[11]

In television and cinema portrayals, men whose work entails making decisions that involve many dollars and many lives ("type A" men) are depicted as predisposed to drop dead from heart attacks brought on by the stress of their powerful positions. Yet a weighty body of literature shows that the most severe job strain is characterized not by authority but rather by high pressure combined with little authority or discretion over use of skills. Men and women working in "high responsibility plus low authority" jobs show significantly elevated rates of myocardial infarction, hypertension, depression, suicide, alcoholism, and gastrointestinal illnesses (Karasek and Theorell 1990). The health status of British civil servants, for example, correlates to their position in the employment hierarchy, and even among the well-educated and well-paid there are incremental differences in health status that parallel job status. Those in the civil service's professional-executive grade have been found to have a significantly higher risk of dying over the course of a decade than their immediate supervisors in the top administrative posts. The professional-executive grade is a perfect fit for the profile of high responsibility/low control positions; these employees are likely to manage large sums of money, big building projects, and extensive human resources, yet they are not the ones who set the policies that establish the parameters within which they must operate (Adler and Corriell 1997; see also Marmot et al. 1997).

Marianne Frankenhaeuser (1991) found that Volvo employees who felt that they could not influence their work conditions and that top management did not listen to what they said reported more somatic symptoms than employees who felt empowered. Moreover, gender rather than occupational status was the best predictor of feelings of authority or absence of authority at work. In self-assessments of symptoms (including gastrointestinal, musculoskeletal, cardiovascular, and mental) the most symptoms were reported by women clerical workers followed by women managers, with men managers and clerical workers reporting the fewest symptoms. Suzanne Haynes (1991) has found that people who work in situations of low job control combined with high job demand are more likely to suffer from gastrointestinal ailments, alcohol-related illnesses, and heart problems. Significantly, many of women's most standard occupations fit this high-strain model. The classic example of a population that suffers from the high responsibility/low authority syndrome is nurses, who are accountable for the very lives of their patients yet lack both authority to order treatment and control over their own work schedules (Coleman and Dickinson 1984). Studies consistently have shown that the health profile of nurses is poor. One study carried out by the U.S. National Institutes for Occupational Safety and Health ranked 130 occupations according to their incidence of mental health problems. Licensed practical nurses, nursing aides, and registered nurses were ranked 3, 10, and 27 respectively (Doyal 1995, 172).

Television stereotypes notwithstanding, these studies suggest that authority and a sense of control enhance health; absence of control detracts from health. Israeli women, like women in other countries, tend to be employed in the kinds of positions in which they have little command over policy, product, or working conditions. But more than that, high responsibility and pressure coupled with low authority seems to characterize not just the work but the entire life situation of Israeli women. Extrapolating from research that examines the health outcomes of employment in high pressure/low control jobs, I suggest that Israeli women are made sick by sustained life experiences of high responsibility (carrying in their bodies the purity and continuity of the collective) coupled with little authority or power.

One of the most obvious indicators of power is political representation, especially at high levels of government. Israel falls behind almost all developed countries in this measure of gendered authority. There have never been more than two women ministers at a time in the Israeli cabinet, and in several cabinets there were none (out of totals of approximately eighteen ministers in each cabinet). The percentage of women Knesset members has not topped 9.1. (The party distribution is uneven: the Orthodox parties usually have no women; most women Knesset members have been from the Labor Party.) One of the best indicators of national authority is membership on the Knesset committees that hold real power to shape Israeli society and determine its future. The Finance Committee has had no women members for most of Israel's history, nor has the all-important Security and Foreign Affairs Committee (Reiss 1998, 52–53). Women do not decide if Israel goes to war or with whom, or how tax money is allocated among the various social, infrastructural, and security needs of the nation. It is difficult to think of a more blatant expression of "low control."

In Israel the top echelons of government and the business sector are intertwined with the top echelons of the IDF—an institution that openly and systematically excludes women from positions of power and prestige, and that valorizes male bodies, male bonding, and male authority (Izraeli 1997). Few Israeli women are company managers. By 1996 women reached a peak of filling approximately 20% of the managerial positions in some fields (Reiss 1998, 47). Even those women who do reach managerial status benefit less from prestige than men: Only half as many women managers as men are given company cars, a significant symbol of status in Israeli culture (48). Being given a company car is both a gesture of respect on the part of the company, and an indicator of mobility, belonging, and independent presence in the public sphere; the car is probably the most important facilitator of bodily autonomy in developed countries.

Approximately half of government employees in Israel are women, yet in the very highest civil service rank (rank 24) there are no women at all; women make up only 7% of the next highest rank (Reiss 1998, 48–49). The percentage of government companies with women directors is minuscule; some companies still have no women directors (50–51). By the late 1990s, the representation of women among Israeli athletes reached 24%. But when we look at who makes decisions about sports—decisions that have an enormous and direct impact on women's bodies—we find that almost no women are members of boards of athletic associations (72).

The gendering of authority in Israeli culture grows and develops over the life courses of individuals. While the most egalitarian elements of the curriculum developed by the Israeli Ministry of Education may be actively implemented only rarely, the official state-produced curriculum does teach that both boys and girls contribute to the Israeli state; the curriculum acknowledges the importance of encouraging both girls and boys to succeed in school and in career; the family and sexuality education programs published by the Ministry of Education present very positive messages regarding girls' and boys' sexuality. Jewish girls study in high school at the same rate as boys, pass their matriculation exams and begin university just as boys do, and by 1996 even more women than men were receiving bachelor and master of arts degrees (see Reiss 1998, 60–63, for statistics on school enrollment). But women make up only 34.7% of university lecturers (the lowest academic rank) and the percentage of women goes down as rank goes up. Women constitute a mere 7.8% of full professors—the rank that confers membership in the university senates, the primary decision-making bodies in Israeli universities (Reiss 1998, 66).

Not even in the arena of life in which Israeli women gain much supposed esteem—natality—do women have significant authority. Women are responsible for producing children, yet the medical system that controls pregnancy, birth, and the health care of children is patriarchal and authoritarian; doctors are paternalistic and women often feel powerless regarding their own health. Contraception (which gives women some measure of autonomy over their own bodies) is not included in the basic basket of services that the government requires health insurers to provide, yet hospital committees that have the power to grant or deny women abortions typically hold women responsible for contraceptive failure, and women who have babies are certainly held responsible for caring for and raising them. Still, women have no authority over the accessibility of contraception, or—and these are probably the more important issues—whether their husbands are willing to cooperate in the use of contraception, whether their communities will look askance at women who limit the number of children they bear, or (for Orthodox women) whether their rabbis will permit the use of contraception at all.

Another authoritarian institution with a large stake in women's bodies is the religious establishment. Rabbis and other "holy men" (such as Rabbi Kaduri, the Baba Sali, the Lubavitcher Rebbe), dead or alive, are leaders in a world in which God is the ultimate authority, rabbis and other holy men share in some of that authority, and women have little authority at all. The typical model of interaction between menstruating, sick, or infertile women and the male rebbe, rabbi, or saint is hierarchical and dogmatic: The holy man gives orders regarding which doctors to consult, which prayers to say, and which *mitzvot* (religious commandments) to observe, as well as when and how to consult, pray, and observe.

Even housework (which in Israel like in most other societies is carried out primarily by women) provides women with a great deal of responsibility but little true authority. Homemakers are expected to soothe and protect childen and husband from the barbs of an outside world over which they themselves have no control, an expectation that is especially poignant for mothers and wives of men in a society in which military duty is an ongoing part of life. Harriet Rosenberg explains that

> Women sometimes experience motherwork, especially in combination with housework and wifework, as exhausting and depressing because they have little scope for real decision-making. In fact, every small decision a woman makes during the day becomes a demand in itself . . . [what to cook, which clothes to wash]. Such pseudochoices have no fundamental impact on the overall structure of the working conditions of domestic labor. They are simply part of the ideology of "freedom of choice" under capitalism which diverts attention away from larger issues by focusing attention on the trivialities of minor consumer choices . . . Women are rarely "their own bosses." (1984, 223)

Not their own bosses at home, rarely the boss in the workplace, never the boss in the IDF, many Israeli women suffer from role overload and role spillover as they juggle employment outside the home with household and family responsibilities (cf. Wortman, Biernat, and Lang 1991). The intensive caretaking that characterizes the years of early parenthood throughout the world is rekindled for Israeli women when their sons enter the IDF. Israeli mothers are likely to bring or send their sons food at their bases, provide laundry services when their sons come home on weekends, and have food waiting for soldier-sons when they arrive (and it is not uncommon for an anxiously awaited son to be held back at the base at the last minute, to decide to visit a friend instead of coming home, or to show up with an unannounced guest or two). But above all, as we will discuss in chapter 3, Israeli mothers carry the burden of worrying while their sons are in the IDF, a burden that takes a significant toll on women's health.

Israeli women not only work outside the home while on average caring for more children than their counterparts in other Western countries, they may also be juggling responsibility for aged, sick, or disabled family members. In the women's health survey conducted through *At* magazine, a third of the women reported that they take care of elderly or infirm family members, a role that most said has a negative impact on their daily functioning (Avgar and Gordon 1997). In another article, Amy Avgar pointed out that,

> Were it not for the role that women play as front-line health care distributors, the formal delivery system would probably be strained beyond capacity. Yet, not only is their social contribution taken for granted by society, but the expertise and experience accrued by women, as informal caregivers, are rarely taken into account by practitioners and policymakers. Consequently, in both formal and informal health care roles, women have little influence over decisions in matters of health—theirs or their family's. (1997, 48)[12]

High responsibility and low authority is a configuration that certainly characterizes women's experiences in many male-dominated contexts. But it seems to me that the idealization of military leaders, great rabbis, and doctors in Israel intensifies that configuration in a way that may particularly detract from women's well-being. Research has shown that poor relations with supervisors, more than with co-workers, tend to be especially deleterious to health: Women who perceive their supervisors as nonsupportive, unfair, and not respectful report more frequent physical and psychological problems. Significantly, the larger the number of supervisors a woman reports to, the more frequent the physical complaints and feelings of anxiety (Swanson et al. 1997, 149). Again extrapolating to Israeli society in general, I suspect that (at least in part) the poor health of Israeli women reflects having to answer to rabbis *and* doctors *and* generals *and* bosses *and* husbands *and* the consumer economy, all of which compete and collude in shifting alliances of power to define and control that most valuable of cultural resources—women's bodies.

What This Book Sets Out to Do

Two intersecting arguments are developed throughout this book. The first is that patriarchy makes women sick. The second is that Jewish Israeli forms of patriarchy make Jewish Israeli women sick in particular ways. I have chosen to focus on issues and institutions that are characteristically Israeli (for example, government encouragement of natality, normalization of militarization, institutionalized role of rabbis) rather than issues like the double workload of paid employment and housework which affect women throughout the world and have been well documented in the scholarly literature. But this choice should not be taken to mean that other patriarchal configurations are less sickening to women.

In crafting this project I decided to limit my discussion to the corporeal experiences of Jewish Israeli women—women whose lives are shaped by their shared citizenship and ethnic location in the Israeli state and by a religious and cultural tradition that has, over a period of thousands of years, constructed very particular sorts of gendered human beings. Christianity and Islam have developed their own gendering patterns and devices which differ in important ways from those of Judaism, and citizenship in the Israeli state has a very different impact upon the corporeal realities of Jewish and Arab women (for example, the state's sponsorship of maternity is meant to encourage Jewish natality, the IDF is meant to protect Jewish "womenandchildren," and only Jewish young women serve in the IDF). Even within the parameters that I have set, the range of corporeal experience is enormous; age, personal inclination, country of origin, class, sexual orientation, and individual life events shape the bodily reality of each woman in unique, dynamic, and multilayered ways. I have tried to do justice to this diversity by devoting half of the chapters of this book to the voices and experiences of individual women; the other chapters focus more on public policy and public discourse.

Contemporary anthropology envisions and describes cultures as constituted by dynamic social processes in which different actors' interpretations of the world become more or less hegemonic in various contexts and at various times. All cultural constructions are contested, including the ones I have described here. In the chapters that follow we will look at the conceptualizations and practices of gendered corporeality that are promulgated by the state and by other powerful institutions, and we will look at the ways in which these conceptualizations and practices are experienced, embraced, and resisted by particular Israeli women.

I have organized this book around the major institutions that shape Israeli women's corporeal experiences. These institutions include motherhood, the media and the consumer economy, the IDF, the medical establishment, the Knesset, and the religious establishment.

Chapter 1 provides background on Israeli national ideology, introducing state discourses through an examination of Knesset debates regarding women's bodies. The specific topics I have chosen to explore are the "demographic problem," monetary grants linked to hospitalization for birthing mothers, and abortion. In all three cases the state declared itself to have legitimate interests in women's bodies, and granted the medical establishment a monopoly on carrying out those interests. Chapter 2 turns from state policies of motherhood to women's maternal experiences. We shall see how motherhood slips out of women's control; the project of maternity seems to unravel in women's hands as representatives of various powerful institutions pull and pick at women's reproductive bodies. Listening to interviews with postpartum women, we hear about their feelings of dependence upon rabbis and doctors, a dependence tied to a sense of mistrust regarding their own bodies' abilities to carry and deliver a healthy child. These themes are then traced through women's experiences of infertility and breastfeeding.

Chapter 3 focuses upon women and the military. In the Israeli context the ideal body is envisioned to be the fighting male body, created through training in weapons and in physical fitness. Within the framework of a conceptual system in which gender is formulated dichotomously and in which gender difference is understood to be essentially physical, women cannot achieve that ideal. The creation of a female body in opposition to the "normative" healthy and strong male body demands that girls and women assimilate unhealthy corporeal expectations. I argue that within the culture of militarization women are construed as "rape-able," in part to legitimate the entire military enterprise. This leads to a more general discussion of rape in Israeli society and a discussion of the illness consequences of living in a culture of gendered violence.

Chapter 4 considers the rhetoric surrounding niddah (menstrual taboos) and immersion in the mikveh (ritual bath). I show that much of this rhetoric constructs women as inherently weak and unhealthy, and in need of ritual attention in order to ameliorate (temporarily) their weakness and poor health. The second part of chapter 4 looks at the experiences of Jewish Israeli brides, who are obligated to immerse in the mikveh whether or not they themselves are religiously observant. This arrangement is a consequence of political compromises in which the state has given the Orthodox rabbinical establishment a monopoly over marriage and divorce. The thrust of this chapter is the symbolic devices that construct female corporeal weakness sometimes even more effectively than more direct techniques of coercion and rational persuasion.

Chapter 5 develops the issue of scrutiny of women's bodies. Beginning with some general comments about the portrayal of women in the Israeli media, the chapter continues with a discussion of Pnina Rosenblum, a beauty queen, glamour girl, cosmetics magnate, and politician who has been called the "breasts of the nation" and the "most typical Israeli woman." The second half of chapter 5 investigates a series of religious conflicts in which scrutinized women's bodies served either as battlefield or as booty. The chapter ends with a discussion of anorexia—the ultimate case of scrutiny and control of women's bodies.

The analysis of Israeli gendering offered in this book is but one of many possible "takes" on gender in Israel. My analysis grew out of involvement in a feminist health activist organization, the Israel Association for the Advancement of Women's Health. Ill health having been my starting point, much of the material presented here emphasizes "negative" aspects of Israeli culture, and I do wish to make clear that I, like other anthropologists and other feminists, also see many dimensions of Israeli culture that are affirming and appreciative of women's experiences. Thus the Conclusion addresses questions of what happens when women resist the gendered structures outlined in the earlier chapters, and points to some of the cultural resources already available to Israeli women.

The relative ease with which I could find most of the data presented in this book gives me a certain cautious optimism. For example, we know about rates of gang rape because there are rape crisis centers in Israel that keep track of calls for help; we know about domestic violence because newspapers consider wife-battering a crime worth reporting rather than the normative right of men to slap around unsatisfactory women. We know about the patriarchal attitudes of certain politicians because there have always been a few strong feminists in the Knesset who have engaged their colleagues in public conversation about women's problems and rights, in the process both raising consciousness and prompting the blatantly sexist retorts that became part of the accessible public record. And we know that Israeli women are sick because Sima and Rachel and Sarah and Mazal and Zehava vociferously complain, and because a growing number of feminist academics, activists, and politicians take those complaints seriously.

Chapter 1

Collective Representations of Motherhood

The "Demographic Problem," Maternity Grants, and Abortion

While they were still some distance from Efrat, Rachel began to give birth and had great difficulty. And as she was having great difficulty in childbirth the midwife said to her, "Don't be afraid, for you have another son." As she breathed her last, for she was dying, she named her son Ben Oni ["son of my sorrow"], but his father named him Benjamin ["son of my right hand"]. So Rachel died and was buried on the way to Efrat, that is Bethlehem. And Jacob set a pillar upon her grave; that is the pillar of Rachel's grave to this day. —GENESIS 35:16–19

Thus says the Lord: A voice is heard in Ramah, lamentation and bitter weeping. Rachel is weeping for her children. She refused to be comforted for her children, because they are not [here]. Thus says the Lord: Keep your voice from weeping and your eyes from tears, for your acts shall be rewarded, says the Lord; and they shall come back again from the land of the enemy. And there is hope for your future, says the Lord, and your children shall come back again to their own border. —JEREMIAH 31:14 ff., in the context of the Babylonian Exile

Looking at the construction of women as mothers in Israeli law, Nitza Berkovitch cites public officials speaking out on motherhood as women's national mission. Parliamentary discussions make it clear: Women should be given equality, treated well, and protected through legislation because women are mothers and mothers are wonderful. In his presentation of the Equal Rights Law back in 1951, Dov Yosef, the Minister of Justice laid the groundwork for contemporary understandings of Israeli womanhood. "Above all, in fulfilling her duty and privilege as a Hebrew mother cherishing the young generation and educating them . . . in all that, the Hebrew woman and mother continues the great tradition of the Israeli heroine" (cited in Berkovitch 1997, 611).

In the same Knesset discussion, Israel's first Prime Minister, David Ben Gurion, also chose to speak about Jewish mothers and mythic heroines rather than about women's rights: "I will talk about my mother, but refer to all mothers. Mother is the most precious person to everyone . . . my mother died when I was ten . . . but still I know that she was the symbol of purity, love, devotion, and nobility" (cited in Berkovitch 1997, 612). Ben Gurion's maternal imagery is deeply embedded in traditional Jewish conceptualizations. His idealized noble mother is a dead mother—harking back to the only Biblical woman who has become the focus of a popular cult in contemporary Israel: Rachel Imeinu, Muter Ruchel, Our Mother Rachel (Sered 1998). The tomb of the Biblical matriarch Rachel, located on the outskirts of Bethlehem, is a focal shrine for women suffering from infertility and difficult pregnancies. In Jewish tradition, Our Mother Rachel, who died in childbirth on the road from Jerusalem to Hebron, endlessly cries over and intercedes on behalf of her children in their Exile. Ben Gurion's language is mythic; his mother is not an agent but a symbol. And the symbolic load she carries is heavy: purity, love, devotion, and nobility.

Public tributes to maternity are among the more poetic expressions of Israeli concern with national survival, population growth, and women's bodies—three themes that have become intertwined in Israeli discourse. The "demographic question" has been raised regularly over the years in the Knesset.[1] The "problem," as it is usually called, has to do with the fact that there are more Arabs than Jews in the Middle East, and that even within Israel the Jewish majority is not as substantial as some might wish. The solution that is generally suggested is for Jewish Israeli women to bear more children. The "demographic problem" and the conscription of women to solve it have constituted a centerpiece of Israeli gendered discourse from the first years of the state and underpin a great many social norms, beliefs, and conventions (some of which are explored in this book).

In order to illustrate the kinds of discourse at work—and the kind of female body that these discourses describe—I turn to one of the many "internal immigration" (*aliya pnimit*) discussions held in the Knesset. On July 10, 1968, Eliezer Shostack (of HaMercaz HaHofshi, the Free Center Party)[2] asked that the Knesset schedule a full-scale debate on the topic of "Government Means for Encouraging Natality in the State." Tying together a range of cultural, political, and economic issues and perching them on the backs (or, more precisely, wombs) of Israeli women, Shostack opened by pointing out that the Six Day War "thank God, [has] changed the entire picture of the country and its population." The problem is that the Six Day War bequeathed on Israel a large Arab population, yet

> the rate of natural growth among our people in Israel is in a dangerous decline. In 1950 the rate of natural growth of our people was twenty-seven to each thousand; in 1965—after fifteen years—the rate dropped to sixteen for each thousand. In

contrast, the rate of natural growth of the population not of our people increased and reached, in the same year . . . forty-six to every thousand. And that was before the Six Day War.

Shostack clarified that among Jews the birth rate differed between the new immigrant population (mostly *Mizrahi*, that is, North African and Asian Jews or Jews of North African or Asian descent) and the veteran population (mostly Ashkenazi, that is, of European Jewish background). New immigrants who had not yet adopted the habits of European Jews, "thank God," had a birth rate of twenty-nine per one thousand. Unfortunately, according to Shostack, that was changing: "And [the new immigrants] also are beginning to get ruined [*l'hitkalkel*]." The longer immigrants are in the country, he said, the lower their natality rate becomes. "It also turns out that the level of education is a factor that detracts rather than encourages. Women without education give birth to six to eight children. The same women from among the immigrants who arrived in Israel, after they learn at schools in Israel, have only two children." Shostack rounded off his remarks with the authority of ancient tradition, reminding the Knesset that the first commandment in the Torah is to be fruitful and multiply (cf. Genesis 1:28). While I doubt that Shostack would like his words summed up in this way, it does seem that he was suggesting that education for women, or at least for Jewish women, is a bad thing for the Jewish collective. In fact, despite idealizations of the mythic Jewish mother, tension between what is good for women and what is good for the state is a theme that reiterates throughout Israeli political discourse.

Prime Minister Levy Eshkol then took the floor and began with an appeal to national consensus, reminding the Knesset that the Jewish people are bereaved after the Holocaust. Therefore, it is important to have children to build up the country. In addition, he counseled that Israel needed more population either from immigration or from natality for the social and economic development of the country. "There is no possibility of high momentum development without human resources. People are producers and consumers." Levy Eshkol thus augmented Shostack's charge to women to lend their bodies to the Jewish national mission and to Torah law, with the additional demand to use their bodies for economic development through the creation of more consumers and producers.

In this chapter I analyze two sets of Knesset debates in which questions of the state and its rights in and over women's bodies were expounded upon. The decisions and laws that ensued from these debates have established institutional frameworks that continue to shape women's lives in the 1990s and beyond. Both in the case of abortion and in the case of maternity grants for women who give birth in hospitals, the Knesset chose to codify what it saw as the national interest in women's bodies by defining women's bodies as likely to need medical treatment and by passing legislation that effectively requires even healthy women to be drawn into the net of the medical establishment for the management of their reproductive lives.

Birth Grants: Multiple Motives

> The Jewish-Israeli female subject is constructed first and foremost, not as an individual or a citizen, but as a mother and a wife. The state, using rhetoric of equality, incorporates the Jewish-Israeli woman via these traditional roles and not through the universal characteristics of citizenship. —Nitza Berkovitch, "Motherhood as a National Mission"

The Knesset has held a series of debates concerning the reasons and conditions for giving new mothers a *ma'anak leda*, a birth grant furnished by the government to cover the cost of childbirth and to allow the mother to purchase necessary equipment for the new baby, and *dmei leda*, a birth allowance that pays women their salary (actually, until recently, 75% of their salary) for a certain period of time following childbirth. (In the Knesset discussions, the two terms sometimes are used interchangeably, but that should not be problematic for our discussion here.) During the 1950s, these debates set out the parameters for the institutionalization of relations between mothers and the state. In the speeches of Knesset members, we discern the origins of Israel's health care system in an Ashkenazi-dominated welfare program that dispensed free medical care along with large doses of paternalism, ethnocentrism, and the belief that medical experts are the only ones who can decide what is "in the best interests" of the patient or birthing woman.

On November 17, 1953, the Knesset addressed the clause of the *Bituah Leumi* (Social Security) Law having to do with the form and amount of financial assistance that the government will give to birthing and new mothers. The proposed policy was to give money only to women who come to hospitals to give birth.[3] Prompting this policy was the enormous influx of North African and Asian immigrants who brought with them childbirth practices at odds with the state's preference for modern, Western medicine. Speakers from various parties addressed the advantages and disadvantages of a number of different proposed means and incentives for encouraging new immigrant women to come to the hospitals for childbirth.

Knesset member Dr. Ben-Zion Harel (of HaZionim HaK'laliyim, a centrist party) explained on behalf of the committee proposing the law:

> We live in a country in which a substantial portion of the inhabitants still are not accustomed to medical care; superstitions still abound in this area among large

parts of the nation, and especially among the women. In these conditions is it possible to give a birth grant and birth allowance without supervision that the birth will at least be carried out by a [licensed] midwife?. . . There are sizable numbers of women who out of superstition don't want to go to a hospital. This particular superstition is especially rampant among a large part of the nation. That is why we must hold to all means of educating and taking care and medical supervision.

Yakov Riftin (of Mapam, United Worker's Party) objected to a clause in the proposed law that would give the government the authority to cancel a woman's right to the birth allowance in part or in full if she had not followed orders regarding medical supervision during pregnancy and birth. Yet even his objection (and Riftin was one of the Knesset members most concerned with women's rights) had nothing to do with women's corporeal autonomy.

There is no disagreement between us that there is a need for medical supervision during pregnancy and birth, but we can't ignore the fact that to bring women to this sort of medical supervision cannot be done by decree but rather by public education. Among our public in Israel there are still backward classes [*sh'chavot m'fagrot*], without enough training. Things that other parts of the public take for granted, these groups do not take for granted. These groups need to slowly acquire concepts and demands that they were not accustomed to in the area of birth and pregnancy. I believe that to punish this population by taking away their birth allowance will not bring those women to a correct understanding of their ability, and their rights as mothers, but will push them even further away from that part of the public characterized by correct civilized achievements.

During the debate, only one Knesset member, Esther Vilenska (of Maki, Israeli Community Party), spoke out in favor of the government's assisting mothers by giving each a sum of money to use as she herself sees fit. All other Knesset members were clear in their conviction that the government should encourage hospital births—that the government knows what is best for women.[4]

The 1953 discussion did not resolve these issues. On June 13, 1955, the Knesset held the first reading of an amendment to the birth grant clause of the Social Security Law. This time the debate was much more complex, drawing on a wider repertoire of discursive stances and institutional interests. Some Knesset members were concerned with the health of women as individuals, others were more concerned about public health, and still others seem to have been most concerned that the birthing woman would survive to bear and raise more children. The "demographic problem" was raised repeatedly, as was the refrain of spreading the "civilized" way of doing things to the "superstitious" masses. And, finally, a number of Knesset members voiced religious concerns and saw the birth grant as a means of encouraging women in Israel to behave in accordance with traditional Jewish models.

The discussion began with Labor Minister Golda Meyerson (Meir) introducing a proposal to double the birth grant for baby items in the case of twins. Although the proposed amendment did not directly address the issue of hospitalization for childbirth, that is what Knesset members chose to focus upon. Hanan Rubin of Mapam pointed out that if a woman does not go to the hospital, which is most likely because of lack of transportation but could also happen for other reasons, she should still receive the entire grant, though, according to the phrasing of the law, she would not. Beba Idelson, a woman Knesset member (of Mapai, Israeli Worker's Party) rejoined that Rubin failed to understand the purpose of the law: to safeguard the health of the mother and child.

> And that is why the Knesset passed a law that says a simple thing: All mothers in labor must give birth in hospitals, for their own good and for the good of their children. That is why the law connects giving the birth grant to a stay in the hospital. The point is that for a woman to give birth in a hospital is a good thing . . . There is no denial of rights in this; there is careful concern for the family.

Ben-Zion Harel added that, "All over the world hospitalization for birthing mothers is an important factor in the framework of public health." Eliezer Shostack also supported the amendment, because of its potential to influence women to have more children. And finally, Shlomo Lorenz of the ultra-Orthodox Agudat Yisrael (Association of Israel Party) explained his point of view:

> The blessing and commandment that come first in our Torah are "Be fruitful and multiply and fill the earth and conquer it." And if during thousands of years, also in difficult conditions, that blessing was found among the Jewish people, then we have before us a difficult paradox—that of all places here in our independent State we are very far from keeping the first of the 613 commandments and we are far from that blessing without which the land cannot be conquered.[5] Encouraging the birth rate is social security and national security of the highest order.

Discussions of the birth grant came up periodically over the years as new concerns entered public consciousness. On October 31, 1994, an amendment was proposed that would give the birth grant to adoptive mothers. The across-the-board support for this amendment, in a Knesset that was bitterly divided over most other issues, sheds light on the strong national consensus regarding the importance of motherhood. One of the most revealing comments was offered by Shaul Yahalom (of Mafdal, National Religious Party), who voiced concern that the feelings of adoptive mothers, who had already suffered for years unsuccessfully trying to conceive, would be hurt if they were to receive a check that says "birth grant." He suggested calling it instead an "adoption grant." His suggestion, well received by other Knesset members, gave public recognition to the social construction of infertility as a terrible, shameful, and national problem.

On June 20, 1995, the question of twins was again on the Knesset floor. Yoram Less of the Labor Party explained that recent increases in numbers of women undergoing fertility treatments have led to more multiple births. "It is unnecessary to point out that a family that, with *mazel tov* [good fortune], has born to them a bigger number of babies, also has a larger load to carry." Two babies are more than twice as much work as one. "If one cries, the other cries too, they need more care, more than three times as much. Whoever has been through these things understands." The goal of the amendment is "that the government should recognize and support those families and give them a larger birth grant than a regular family receives when they raise one child." Less continued, "That family—I should say that happy family, happy times three and happy times four—will receive a larger birth grant to help them raise their children . . . We absolutely cannot relate to fertility treatments as being a luxury or indulgence." Not a single member of the Knesset spoke out to question whether the government should encourage high-priced and invasive fertility treatments that may harm women's bodies and that all too often result in multiple births of underweight babies or of babies with other health problems.[6]

Subsequent speakers made it clear that their primary concern was not for the harried mother of quadruplets. Uzi Landau of the Likud asserted that the government should do what it could to encourage the birth rate. "I wish to emphasize this especially within the Jewish sector. We talk about the demographic danger . . . the demographic balance between Arab citizens of Israel and Jewish citizens is changing for the worse for the Jews."

And finally the Knesset heard from Yosef BaGad (an Orthodox Knesset member of the very right-wing Moledet [Homeland] Party) who asked for an additional three months of paid maternity leave (birth allowance) for each additional child in the same birth. Bringing familiar mythic discourse into the Knesset debate, BaGad declared: "At least let us unite in a national consensus [on this matter]. As Rachel said to Our Father Jacob: 'Give me sons, and if not,' God forbid [*halila*] 'I will die. Give me sons.' Give me the possibility of raising children for the State of Israel."

Aborting the National Mission

Israel's current abortion law is the product of compromise among political parties representing some very diverse value systems. In this case, as in others that we will see, women's bodies served as a convenient site for the struggle to define the culture of the state. That the actual issue at hand had to do with the regulation of women's bodies allowed unusually complex intertwining of both direct (legislative) and symbolic (discursive) corporeal control.

Conceptualizations and practices of abortion hold extraordinary power to construct particular sorts of female bodies. Legalization of abortion can construct an autonomous female body, or alternatively, a female body understood to be available for limitless sexual activity or services. Prohibitions against abortion forcibly construct maternal bodies or, alternatively, criminalized bodies. In either case, the implications for women's health are severe. In the Israeli situation, as we shall see, abortion is restricted—neither illegal nor universally available—leading to the construction of a rhetoricized, scrutinized, medicalized female body.

The Knesset Debate

In line with my understanding that discourse creates corporeal experience, I begin with an analysis of a debate in the Knesset in 1976. Abortion had not previously been conspicuous on the Israeli public agenda. By looking at what was said, and by whom, we can see how certain conceptualizations of the state, God, and gender shaped Israel's first official abortion conversation, a conversation that led to a particular corporeal reality.

At the first reading of an amendment to the Law of Punishments in the Matter of Termination of Pregnancy (January 27, 1976), rationale for a proposed legislative change was presented by Haike Grossman (Mapam, United Workers Party) chair of the Knesset committee for public services. Grossman explained that a 1936 British law prohibiting abortion was still the law of the land in Israel, but social realities had changed and many women in fact were having abortions. Neither the 1936 law nor any other coherent policy was being enforced, and women had no choice but to pay dearly both financially and physically for illegal abortions. While Grossman herself would have liked to see abortion made fully legal and available for women who wished to terminate pregnancies, in order to settle this important matter the Knesset committee had come up with a compromise that would allow abortion on three grounds: If the pregnancy endangers the life or health of the woman, if the pregnancy endangers the life or health of the fetus, and for socio-cultural reasons (including rape, incest, marital status, economic distress). Grossman pointed out that those who oppose allowing abortion in cases of socioeconomic need may not understand the relationship between social distress, psychological distress, and physical illness. "If a woman comes and protests [*kovelet*] that she takes care of a large number of children in conditions of difficult distress and truly has no strength to bring another child into the world, then refusing to allow her to terminate the pregnancy can sentence the woman and her household to emotional and bodily harm." Moreover, Grossman explained, citing "Professor Vinik, Director of Talbiah Psychiatric Hospital" (and thus invoking an authority greater than her own): "If the woman is in an emotional condition that does not allow her to respond to the needs of the child, there is a large danger that the child will not develop emotionally into a healthy person."

In the proposal presented by Grossman, the mechanism for obtaining an abortion would be a two-member committee consisting of a gynecologist and a social worker, public health nurse, or another doctor; both members of the committee would be chosen by the woman herself. Grossman explained that this committee was necessary so that the amendment would pass, but it had an additional advantage in that "it will give legitimacy that has important implications for women from environments of economic and social distress, and especially in cases in which they are considered to be owned by their husbands [*kinyan bidei ba'aleihen*]." In short, Grossman (a savvy politician) chose to frame the amendment that would legalize abortion as a bureaucratic measure designed to protect the health of women and children. Without the state's institutionalizing and supervising abortion, women's health would suffer from unscrupulous or incompetent abortion providers, from endless childbearing and rearing, and from their low position among "certain" ethnic groups.

After Grossman spoke, debate immediately shifted to the question of women and the national responsibility to bear children. The first respondent to the proposal was Geula Cohen of the Likud who voiced her strong objection to the proposed law on demographic grounds. Most other speakers agreed with Cohen about the "demographic problem," yet occasional alternative voices were heard. Shulamith Aloni (of Tnuah l'Zechut HaEzrach, Civil Rights Party) declared, "I want to prevent the kind of situation that I have heard about. A woman with three children goes to the doctor and asks for contraception and he tells her, 'Madam, not yet. You need first to have more children, for ideological reasons.'" And in words even stronger and more overtly feminist than Aloni's, Meir Pa'il (of Moked, "Focus" Party) called out: "A woman isn't a national birth machine. She is a human being."

The objection to the proposed law that was voiced most frequently during the debate was that abortions cause infertility. Menahem Yedid (Likud) opposed the law "for reasons of the woman's health, her children's health, and my conscience." He explained,

We must not forget that in every abortion there is a danger to the woman and to her future health. And thus in each and every case, before the woman takes on herself this dangerous step, there must be a clear diagnosis regarding what is preferable and what is more dangerous, and it is necessary to know the medical implications and the damage to her health.

Yedid quoted doctors who had told him that abortion is traumatic to the woman's body because it stops hormonal processes, that women who have had abortions have a higher rate of bleeding and vomiting in the first trimester of subsequent pregnancies and a higher rate of complications at birth, and "the rate of death in the first few weeks of life is three or even four times higher among babies whose mothers have had an abortion than among those who never have." Linking medical paternalism to a nationalist and religious mission, Yedid clarified that the issue at stake was not merely the well-being of the woman herself: "We must remember that only a healthy mother can function and run a household and educate her children as is fitting and suitable for a mother in Israel." That is why, "out of responsibility for the fate of the nation and belief in the future of Eretz Yisrael . . . I will vote against the law."

Despite his disapproval of abortion (at least for Jewish Israeli women), Yedid was a politician and a realist and understood that the proposed amendment would pass in one form or another, given the Labor Party's majority in the Knesset. Thus he also devoted words to ensuring that even if abortion were to become legal, women would not have true autonomy in the matter. He suggested that instead of one doctor and another advisor both chosen by the woman seeking an abortion (as per the proposed amendment), the abortion committee should consist of two doctors and a social worker, all from an approved list (the woman could, however, choose a rabbi instead of the social worker). In words that sum up almost all of the discursive positions expressed by the various parties, "And so the [abortion] committee [will] set principles and put an emphasis upon giving permission according to clear criteria, *according to the woman's good and NOT according to her wishes*" (my emphasis).

Other Knesset members agreed that it would be intolerable for a woman to do what she wants with her body. Spelling out the diverse institutions that compete for control over women's bodies, Aharon Abuhatzeira (of Hazit Datit Leumit, National Religious Front) declared:

I am full of respect and admiration for the year of women's equality [1976]. I am willing that women should have any rights in the world that they want, but one thing just cannot be: that a pregnant woman decides for herself when to have an abortion. According to the proposed law she must ask the doctor, the family doctor, the social worker—but she does not need to ask her husband.

Adding further complexity to the Knesset debate was an ongoing undercurrent of ethnic politics. During the January 1976 debate, Ora Namir spoke touchingly about the difficult social and economic conditions of large families in Israel,

> especially for women who can't afford to go to the doctor to get contraception, and even worse, whose backgrounds didn't make them conscious of family planning . . . And there still are many women, very many, who are in a situation of constant pregnancy, women who at age twenty-seven, twenty-eight, twenty-nine are mothers to eight children, or nine or ten. And they are used up, burnt out, exhausted, sad, apathetic, sick. And the yoke of raising the children and educating them falls on their shoulders alone, because the husband spends most of the hours of the day, and often the night as well, outside of the house and family framework, involved in various strange occupations, and often is unaware and irresponsible about carrying the financial burden.

The overwhelmingly Ashkenazi Knesset did not need to have the "backgrounds" spelled out for them—everyone knew Namir was talking about Israel's North African and Asian (Mizrahi) Jewish population.

In the next round of debate on the proposed amendment (held on February 10, 1976), the ethnic cards were laid on the table and named for what they were. Knesset member Abuhatzeira explained why he opposed the clause that would allow abortion for socioeconomic reasons. This clause, "according to Ora Namir's own words," was aimed primarily at the large, poor, non-Ashkenazi families with whom Abuhatzeira identified and whom he had set out to represent. Arguing that the need for such a clause represents the failure of Israel's social and economic programs, he clarified that,

> It is not directed toward those who have one or two children, it is not directed toward women who want an abortion because they do not want more children. It is directed against large families. I say it strongly that this clause is directed to prevent large families, because the state is not able to solve the problems of these families . . . Gentlemen [*sic*] and members of the Knesset, I have heard social workers and other people say to mothers, "For what have you brought this child into the world if you aren't able to support him out of your own money?" And that is [exactly] what you are doing!

Well aware of the coercive efforts of the Ashkenazi elite to socialize new immigrants into "modern" and "hygienic" practices, Abuhatzeira interpreted the liberalized abortion law as actually decreasing free choice for North African and Asian families: "The social worker will dictate [*machtiva*] to the woman to have an abortion."

Abuhatzeira's critique of the ethnocentric social policies of the Ashkenazi political elite reveals the interpenetration of ethnic and gender hierarchies:

Women are disprivileged but so are Mizrahi men. The men he represents feel that they do not have "equal rights" in Israel's democratic society: "I understand that those who want this law see in it a guarantee of equal rights for women. Please, I want equal rights also for the husband."

Few Knesset members even acknowledged Abuhatzeira's comments or concerns. In fact, my sense is that his concerns were incomprehensible to most of the Knesset. Yet his concerns were and are those of large segments of Israel's "traditional" or *masorati*, primarily North African, population, the population that made Shas (Sephardi Torah Guardians) the third largest political party in Israel with seventeen seats in the 1999 Knesset elections. Abuhatzeira knew where he stood vis-à-vis the Knesset: When one Knesset member yelled at him: "What kind of logic is this?" he answered, "The logic of most of the public, and not of most of the Knesset."

Zerah Warhaftig (of Hazit Datit Leumit, National Religious Front), like Abuhatzeira, objected to the husband not having a role in the approval process:

> What kind of *sh'lom bayit* [conjugal harmony] will it bring, how many families can it shake up and destroy when suddenly one day the husband comes home and the wife is no longer pregnant, and he didn't know? How many families will be destroyed? . . . Gentlemen [*sic*], I refer you to a saying of our Sages. "Three partners create a child: the woman, the husband, and above all—the Holy One Blessed Be He." And you want to throw two out of that partnership. You want to throw out the husband and the Holy One Blessed Be He.

Knesset members from the Orthodox religious parties linked the proposed abortion legislation to ancient national myths. Pinhas Scheinman (of Hazit Datit Leumit), for example, described the proposed law as a *g'zera* or decree worse than that of Pharaoh who wanted to kill only the Israelite boys, whereas abortion would kill both boys and girls. This *g'zera* for Scheinman was tied not only to the distant national past, but also to the more recent past and to the demographic present—"the Holocaust in which one million children were killed." Noting that the number of Arabs was increasing faster than the number of Jews, he asked, "Don't we know that every [Jewish] birth is an addition to national security?"

The mythic motif was developed further by Shlomo Yaakov Gross (of Hazit Datit Toranit, Religious Torah Front), who added his own gendered spin:

> When the Jews lived in terrible conditions and were enslaved in Egypt, Miriam [the sister of Moses] understood that it was crucial to think about the birth rate, continuing the generations. And she advised her father to return to his wife [the men of Israel, according to the midrash, lost the will to reproduce under slavery]. That is not how the women Knesset members of today act. Miriam said: "Although

I live a life of sorrow, we must not stop the birth rate of the nation." And Amram [Moses' father] listened to his daughter, and returned his wife, and the redeemer of Israel was born, Moshe Rabeinu [Moses].

Gross continued, "When Israel was enslaved in Egypt the women went into the fields and seduced their husbands so that they could give birth in Egypt, in the most terrible conditions . . . Miriam saw the future of the People of Israel from a different perspective than that of today's women Knesset members. In the merit of the women of Israel, Israel was redeemed [from Egypt]."

In this discursive banquet, medical, religious, demographic, nationalist, mythic, ethnic, and economic discourses engage and disengage repeatedly, constructing a female body that is the legitimate object of multi-institutional scrutiny. What I find most interesting in the Knesset debate is the absence of the issue central in the abortion debate in the United States—the fetus. With the exception of one or two Knesset members who shouted out "it's murder" (comments that no one else related to), the speakers focused on women's bodies and the needs of the state.[7]

One point puzzled me the first few times that I read through the record of the lengthy debates: Several Knesset members who opposed the amendment seemed to assume that it would lead to mandatory abortion (rather than freedom to choose to have or not to have an abortion). Repeatedly, Knesset members voiced concern that the proposed amendment will mean that women will *have* to have abortions, that someone or some institution will force abortions on women. Where was this argument coming from? Did those who opposed the amendment willfully misinterpret both its actual wording and Haike Grossman's very clear introductory explanation? Or could it be that the notion of a woman freely choosing what to do with her own body was incomprehensible to many members of the Knesset?

The gendered conceptual schema underlying the Knesset debate was comprised of competing authoritarian institutions vying for control of women's bodies. Thus if, for example, religion were to relinquish control, the medical establishment would take control; if the medical establishment were to relinquish control, the North African family with its "primitive" birth customs would take control; if the husband were to relinquish control, the state would take control. With the exception of a very few speakers (Marcia Freedman, Meir Pa'il, Shulamith Aloni) the question that was debated was *which* institution should hold power over women's bodies, and not *whether* any institution at all should hold such power. For most of the speakers, the question of women's rights was irrelevant.

While I think it is reasonable to interpret the Knesset debate over abortion as an interinstitutional dispute, one institution, to my reading, held a privileged position throughout: the medical establishment. Doctors, medical specialists, and medical considerations were mentioned by almost all of the speakers, whether for or against the amendment. This kind of discursive borrowing (or infiltration) reveals the power of one institution to frame the discourse of another. But more than that, the privileged place of the medical establishment in the discursive arena became institutionalized in the current system of three-member abortion granting committees in which physicians outnumber social workers two to one.

The dominance of medical experts and formulations in the Knesset debate led to an abortion law that makes women sick. It does so by defining a woman who wants an abortion as ill and in need of "cure" by two doctors. And indeed, legal abortions in Israel are highly medicalized, performed under general anesthesia in hospitals where women are kept under hospital surveillance for at least twenty-four hours after the procedure. When in 1979 the Knesset voted to amend the 1976 law by removing the clause in the law that allowed abortions for social and economic reasons, medical conceptualizations truly emerged victorious. Consistently, since 1979, the most heavily used clause—invoked in approximately half of abortion requests—has been pregnancy outside of marriage (Israel Central Bureau of Statistics 1998). In other words, despite the fact that half of abortions are requested for reasons that do not seem to require an expert medical opinion (marital status), doctors hold the power to approve or reject *all* abortion applications. This institutional twist enhances the authority of the medical establishment enormously—constructing it as adjudicator of public morality—at the same time that it defines women's "non-normative" sexual behavior as an illness.

Abortion Committees: Women Examined

> God speaks to Moses to say to the children of Israel. "Should any man among you find that his wife has gone astray and betrayed him and some man had lain with her sexually . . . and she was not caught. And he is then possessed by jealousy and she is defiled or he is possessed by jealousy and she is not defiled. Then the man should bring his wife to the priest . . . and the priest will place the woman before the Lord and uncover the woman's head [and administer the oath and the bitter water]."
>
> —Numbers 5:11 ff.

The state's vested interest in women's bodies is ritually reenacted at every inquisitory meeting of the committees empowered to grant or deny abortions. These committees hold mandated authority to decide which women, and under what circumstances, will be permitted to terminate their pregnancies.

Yael Yishai describes four models of abortion policies employed by Western states in the second half of the twentieth century. The first of these is facilitation, found for example in Sweden, where the state funds and makes abortions available to all women who wish to terminate pregnancies. The second model is restriction, for example in Ireland, where the state (often for religious reasons), prohibits abortion under all, or almost all, circumstances. The third model, the American one, is hindrance—abortion is legal but expensive, difficult to come by, or in some way obstructed by the state or by other powerful institutions. The final model, the one found in Israel, is what Yishai calls intrusion. In this model the state is a major player in each and every abortion decision; by requesting an abortion a woman effectively turns her body over to state scrutiny.

My discussion in this section draws upon research carried out by Delila Amir and Orly Biniamin, who interviewed twenty-nine social workers serving on thirteen of the nineteen abortion approval committees functioning in Israel at the time of their study (1986–1988). According to Amir and Biniamin, although it is not required by law, women requesting abortions are routinely required to meet with a social worker prior to appearing before the committee. They also are told to fill out a detailed questionnaire covering many aspects of their lives and reproductive histories. "Nearly half the social workers reported that they found it important to *examine* the details of the abortion candidate's life, the circumstances of the specific pregnancy and the reasons that it is unwanted" (1992, 14; all emphases mine). In eleven of the thirteen committees, all abortion candidates are required to appear physically before the committee, even though the law demands only that the committee meet with women for whom the requested abortion was *not* approved. Although the law neither requires nor even mentions it, in the context of their appearance before the committee, women are asked questions and then "educated" about the use of contraception. "In this forum, intimate details of her life are again *exposed* and she has to repeat her description of the circumstances of the pregnancy and the reasons for its being defined as 'unwanted'" (14). "The *probing for information* usually focuses on the circumstances under which the pregnancy developed" (15). A social worker explained that, "She [the candidate] must also undergo a gynecological *examination* because it is her pregnancy, and she must take responsibility for it" (15). In Amir and Biniamin's description of the approval process, the word *examine* is used repeatedly: "The social worker *examines* the extent of the woman's determination to forgo the pregnancy" and "she *examines* the candidate's eligibility" (15). Social workers ask for details having to do with the woman's sexual behavior. "If the woman doesn't cooperate,' says one social worker, 'I explain to her that for her own good, it is best that she tell the whole picture'" (16).

In line with Foucault's ideas about power and knowledge, Amir and Biniamin see the approval procedure as a control mechanism. "The abortion candidate is subjected to intimate personal exposure in the context of a threat that the abortion will be denied if she holds back information. This is a clear case of 'discourses concerning sex . . . as the exercise of power itself,'" they wrote, quoting Foucault. The ritual aspect of the approval process becomes even clearer when we understand that almost all requests for abortions are granted. "The low rate of refusals underscores [that] . . . it is the right to choose, and not the right to an abortion, which is taken away from the Israeli woman" (20–21). In fact, social workers explain that they almost always encourage the committees to grant first requests. Subsequent requests, on the other hand, are sometimes denied as a punishment for disregarding the committee's advice on the proper use of contraception (19).

In short, not only is Israel's abortion law framed in such a way as to demand a certain degree of scrutiny of women who request abortions, but the actual implementation of the law involves further elaboration of detailed and ritualized examination of women's bodies, motives, and souls. The near negligible protest regarding the psychically intrusive and physically invasive scrutiny of women's bodies suggests that this sort of scrutiny, in some way, is experienced as fitting a broadly agreed upon meta-discourse of women's bodies exemplified perhaps in the Biblical "bitter waters" test described in the epigraph to this section. The examination of the woman requesting an abortion (ostensibly to see whether she fits the legal requirements and to check whether she is innocent or guilty of the crime of the misuse of contraception) is a prime example of "legitimate" scrutiny of women's bodies as part of larger processes of gendered corporeal control.

Nothing seems to raise the ire of abortion committee members more than women who refuse to follow their "good" advice concerning contraception. In other words, the "bad" woman is one who exercises agency (albeit the not very productive agency of rejecting contraceptive devices) and thus resists her construction as an object of state-defined sexual hygiene. In fact however, one suspects that the real competition is not as much *with* the woman as *over* the woman: between the patriarchal state that demands compliance with its notions of appropriate sexuality and the patriarchal husband, boyfriend, or other man who demands unrestricted access to a woman's body.

Right to Life, Israeli-style

During the past decade the abortion discourse in Israel, although still rather low-key, has begun to incorporate the American Christian rhetoric of "right to life." Yet even the "right to life" typically is presented more as part of a larger program encouraging women's maternity than as a theological program. We shall look here at the anti-abortion rhetoric that recently has become popular in Israel, promulgated for the most part by an organization named Efrat.

Efrat reaches out to pregnant women, offering them financial and social support if they will agree to carry their pregnancies to term. Efrat has a Web site, gives lectures, provides free medical counseling, and produces numerous pamphlets, which are distributed in hospitals, the IDF, schools, and other public forums. Several of Efrat's pamphlets display pictures of "Efrat's children"—attractive, smiling children who were "saved" by Efrat. A popular picture, included in several pamphlets, shows a demonstration of "Efrat's children" held in front of the Knesset; an Israeli flag is waving overhead, visually asserting the association between fertility and nationalism. In an effort to enlist men in the project of persuading women to carry pregnancies, the cover of one Efrat pamphlet shows a happy father holding a cute toddler.

One popular pamphlet,[8] entitled "The Price for an Instant," is written in the form of an open letter from a mother who after many years of secrecy has decided that she must reveal to her teenage daughter why she is an only child. It turns out that the mother became pregnant as a teenager, her boyfriend discarded her, and she had an abortion. Following years of depression and misery she met a kind man and married, and wanted more than anything to start a family. But she could not conceive, and suffered more than nine years of infertility. "When I finally told my secret to the doctor, I heard from him that there is a direct connection between the abortion I had and my condition." After many painful and expensive tests and treatments, doctors told her she probably would not be able to have children. "I finally understood that because I had not stood up for myself and been strong enough [to resist the pressure of the boyfriend and her family to have an abortion], I endangered my future as a mother forever." During the years of fertility treatments she met other women with the same story. "I saw the suffering of women who had undergone an abortion and now are willing to undergo seven hells in order to hear the great news that they are pregnant. They are desperate to hug a child in their arms, but there isn't one."

Conspicuous in this pamphlet is the framing of the abortion discourse in health and medical terms. Her "punishment" for having an abortion was infertility; salvation came from the doctors who treated her. Efrat—an organization with mainly Orthodox members—could have chosen many other discursive techniques, yet wisely chose this one that resonates so well in Israeli culture. Efrat's lecturers and writers assume (probably correctly) that the threat of barrenness will be especially effective for discouraging Israeli women from choosing abortion. As the Biblical epigraphs at the beginning of the next chapter show, this threat is well grounded in Jewish culture.

The inspiration behind Efrat is Dr. Eli Schussheim, an Orthodox physician who has the ears of several Knesset members. He has written a booklet on marriage that features a section entitled "Health and Beauty for the Woman," in which he explains—with all of the authority of his medical degree—that,

> The happiness that comes from having children strengthens the emotional health of the person and has a positive influence on physical health. The absence of these elements, because of failure to fulfill the natural function of the family, can result in absence of satisfaction, in stress and tension that harm the emotional health of the person and so have a bad influence on the physical health as well. There are those who are concerned that bearing many children causes damage to the woman. But reality proves that the opposite is true. The facts prove that mothers of many children, who run their lives according to the biological nature of bearing children, are emotionally healthy and physically strong.

The next section of the booklet turns the heat up another notch: The reader is confronted with pictures tracing the development of an attractive fetus. One page shows the fetus at two-week stages and bears the handwritten caption: "Mommy, look, I'm already big"—an image common in antichoice literature in the United States.

The idea that the fetus is a full human being has been gaining some ground in Israel recently. In late 1998, Deputy Health Minister Shlomo Beniziri (of Shas, Sephardi Torah Guardians) ordered the publication of a booklet with pictures of cute babylike fetuses and the claim that all abortion is murder. Fifteen thousand copies were sent to hospitals to be given to every woman who requests an abortion. The Minister of Health, Joshua Matza, eventually suspended distribution, but he did not order the recall of the copies that were already sent out (*Jerusalem Post*, January 29, 1999; byline Esther Hecht).

The newspaper *Yerushalayim* reported on July 18, 1997, a special ritual to exorcise spirits (*gerush shedim*) from the bodies of women who have had abortions (the word used is *happalot*, which includes both abortions and miscarriages in Hebrew) to be held at Yeshivat HaShalom. "The head of the Yeshiva, a kabbalist by the name of Rabbi David Batzri, had also announced a kabbalistic ritual of spiritual mending [*tikkun n'fashot*] for the fetuses that were aborted/miscarried." The ritual was planned for the seventeenth day of the Hebrew month of Tammuz, a traditional fast day in memory of the destruction of the Temple in Jerusalem. In Jewish belief, the Temple was destroyed because of the spilling of blood, a behavior repeated in our day, according to Rabbi Batzri, in the thousands of abortions performed in Israel each year. In addition to prayers, shofars would be blown to exorcise the spirits in the bodies of the women who had abortions. Rabbi Batzri explained that according to the Mishnah (an ancient compendium of Jewish law) a woman who had an abortion is supposed to fast for three and a half years, but since that is not possible nowadays it is enough for these women to fast only on the day of the ceremony, and then give one shekel (about twenty-five cents) to charity each day for three and a half years. In the ritual described by this well-known kabbalist, I am particularly struck by the way in which women's bodies are drawn into the collective narrative of the destruction of the Temple in a role that metaphorically attributes national disaster to women's bodies. I am equally struck by the effective way in which Rabbi Batzri has encouraged women to think about their corporeal pathology every single day while they give one shekel to charity.

Chapter 2

The Reproductive Body

Pregnancy, Birth, Infertility, and Breastfeeding

And God remembered Sarah as He had foretold, and God did to Sarah as He had said. And Sarah conceived and bore a son for Abraham in his old age, at the time that God had spoken.
—Genesis 21:1

And Isaac prayed to God concerning his wife because she was barren and God answered his prayer and Rebecca his wife conceived. —Genesis 25:21

And God saw that Leah was hated and he opened her womb but Rachel was barren. Then Leah conceived and bore a son and she called him Reuven because she said, "God has seen my misery and my husband will love me now. . . . " Now when Rachel saw that she bore Jacob no children she became jealous of her sister and she said to Jacob, "Give me children or else I die." Then Jacob's anger burned against Rachel and he said, "Am I in the place of God who has withheld from you the fruit of the womb?" —Genesis 29:31–32 and 30:1–2

And to Hannah he [Elkana] gave a twofold portion because he loved Hannah and God had shut up her womb . . . And as time had passed Hannah conceived and bore a son and she called him Sh'muel, "He is lent to me from God". . . And the woman tarried and nursed her son until he was weaned and she brought him up with her when he was weaned . . . and she brought him to God's house in Shilo. —1 Samuel 1:5, 20, 23–24

Multiple Models of Childbirth

This chapter explores how cultural conceptualizations of the maternal body are assimilated by individual Israeli women. At least four distinct models of fertility and childbirth operate among Jews in Israel today: the Western medical model, the formal Jewish model, folk-religious models, and more recently introduced natural childbirth models (cf. Topley 1974 on Hong Kong). All shape women's experiences of pregnancy, birth (in)fertility, breastfeeding, and baby care through representatives or agents who draw women into relationships with external sources of authority. Doctors, midwives, prepared childbirth class instructors, rabbis, circumcisers, and older relatives all have stakes in the maternal body.

I met the women whose experiences we will hear in this chapter in the course of fieldwork that I carried out in 1988 and 1989 on the maternity ward of a Jerusalem hospital, Misgav Ladach. The project was designed to shed light on how women experience and interpret the process of becoming mothers. Misgav Ladach Hospital, primarily a maternity hospital, is known throughout Israel for its personalized approach to childbirth and expressed support for natural childbirth. Husbands are encouraged to remain with their wives during the birth, and the hospital usually allows women to bring personal items such as pictures, tape players, and religious objects into the birthing rooms. Other Israeli hospitals have recently somewhat shifted their childbirth policies to bring them more into line with the policies already instituted by Misgav Ladach in the 1980s, yet strict medical control over birthing women continues to be the norm at Misgav Ladach and throughout Israel.[1]

The bulk of the data were collected through wide-ranging interviews with women resting in their beds after having delivered. In the course of the study I spoke to close to one hundred women, and despite the many distractions on a maternity ward, managed to conduct fairly complete interviews with fifty-five. Our conversations covered obstetrical history, feelings about and description of the pregnancy, birth and postpartum period, and secular and religious rituals surrounding pregnancy, birth, and the newborn baby. All of the women had given birth during the previous few hours or days to live babies. The women were a mixed population in terms of age (from twenty to forty-one), ethnic background (American, Israeli born of European ancestry, Israeli born of North African ancestry, Israeli born of Asian ancestry, North African, Asian, European and South American), education (ten years to eighteen years), obstetrical history, and number of previous children (from none to nine). The Misgav Ladach women are not fully representative of Israel's childbearing population; most notably, American-born women are overrepresented and secular Israeli-born women of Ashkenazi backgrounds are underrepresented.[2] Because post-caesarian women spend more days in the hospital than women who have had vaginal deliveries, I suspect that post-caesarian women are also overrepresented.[3]

The Medical Model, Israeli-style

Eighteen years ago, when I lay in labor in Soroka Hospital in Beer Sheva, another woman in labor on the other side of the partition to my left was shrieking in pain. A male doctor yelled at her: "Do you know why there is a [specialty of] women's doctor [gynecologist in Hebrew is *rofe nashim*—"women's doctor"] and no men's doctor? Because being a woman is a disease." Not a single midwife objected to this. Two years later, when I was in the hospital following the birth of my second child, one male doctor was smoking during the doctors' morning tour of the ward. When I told him this is outrageous in a hospital, he said, "Are you a teacher? It shows." Again, not a single colleague of his responded. —Leah Shakdiel

Nearly all Israeli women give birth in hospitals. This is a matter in which the Israeli state has a self-declared stake: In a hugely successful effort to encourage women to give birth in the hospital rather than at home, a *ma'anak leda* or birth grant from the government covers all hospital costs and even includes a monetary gift for the mother. In addition to hospital care, almost all Israeli women visit doctors at some point in their pregnancies, and prenatal care is easily available and provided virtually for free by the state.

As in the United States, clinic and hospital doctors espouse a medically oriented model of pregnancy and childbirth (cf. Martin 1987).[4] This hierarchical model, treating women and babies as passively dependent upon active, knowledgeable physicians, focuses on the physical and often pathological aspects of birth. An Israeli study conducted among postpartum women in 1995 found that many of the common hospital procedures (including shaving pubic hair, use of monitors, induction of labor, attachment of an IV line, and caesarian sections) are often—in one third to one half of all cases—carried out without the birthing woman's participating in the decision (Zalcberg et al. 1999, 12–13).

Certain of the common medical practices during childbirth actually construct women to be sick. For example, it is the policy at many Israeli hospitals to perform an episiotomy cut on all primipara (first birth) women. I see this policy as a cultural practice that constructs sick female bodies in the double sense of asserting that women cannot "naturally" succeed in birthing their own babies, and of directly causing women a great deal of pain and discomfort during the immediate postpartum period, a time when they are crystallizing their identities and self-images as mothers.

In the Israeli version of the medical model of childbirth, midwives play a pivotal part. Unless a birthing woman has chosen to hire a private doctor (and few do), uncomplicated births are attended by women midwives, some of whom have more and some of whom have less affinity for the strictly medical model of childbirth. The way the system works is that several midwives are on duty during each shift, and laboring and birthing women will be seen by whomever happens to be on duty. When one shift ends, the next roster of midwives takes over. While there are many wonderful and caring midwives, in many other cases midwives neither sit with laboring women nor give women information that might help them feel more in control and able to make informed decisions. In general, the midwife comes in from time to time to check the "progress" of labor and possibly to offer pain medication or a brief exhortation to "relax" or "calm yourself down."[5]

Several women I interviewed told me that they had screamed more than necessary during labor in order to elicit attention from the midwife; others told me that they made an effort to be extra nice to the midwives in order to make sure that they would get help when they needed it. Most laboring women come to perceive the midwives as authority figures in much the same way that doctors are authority figures: They keep themselves physically separate from the laboring women, periodically making definitive pronouncements on the "progress" of the labor. Knowing that a midwife will spend extended time only with women who have "real" problems may tend to set up situations in which women feel compelled to be sick during labor.

One midwife explained to me that she must use authoritarian tactics when the birthing woman is not sufficiently "cooperative" (her word). "When the woman is thrashing around my more effective strategy to calm her is to scare her a bit [by saying]: 'If you continue, you will harm your child' . . . There is also my fear as a midwife that I cannot help or deal with women who are really thrashing around." Elizabeth Grosz has argued that medicalization has the effect of making a "body pliant to power" (1993, 199). Women giving birth in Israeli hospitals know that if something "goes wrong" (a vague and omnipresent danger) or if labor does not progress "quickly enough" (again, a vague danger), a doctor will be called in to administer medication or perform surgery. Some midwives hold out the promise of a doctor coming "to check in on you" (either as a threat or as a reward) as a means of enlisting laboring women's cooperation. This discursive technique, reminiscent of "Wait until your father gets home," reinforces gender hierarchies grounded in unequal access to power and prestige.

The role of midwives in Israeli hospitals is congruent with the role of social workers on abortion committees and (as we shall see later on) with the role of attendants at ritual baths (mikvehs). These are professionally trained women who represent male-dominated establishments to other women; they serve as gatekeepers to the goods and services owned or controlled by a male-dominated institution and required or desired by women clients; and they share with their female clientele the uncomfortable status of holding heavy responsibility without real authority. It is often the case that midwives deflect a great deal of the anger that would have been directed at the (usually male) doctors they represent. Midwives in Israeli hospitals have no authority over policies on the use of fetal monitors, unconventional postures for giving birth, or deciding whether or not to induce labor, yet they must represent and justify these policies to birthing women—even when in particular cases the policy seems to the midwife not to be in the best interests of the patient. Similarly, although Israeli hospitals have fairly firm protocols regarding when midwives may or must call in doctors, patients tend to believe that midwives can choose whether birthing women will see a doctor or not, and midwives are the ones blamed by laboring women for not being helpful or caring about their pain.[6] The high visibility of midwives enhances the prestige and mystique of (the predominantly male) physicians by exempting them from the nitty-gritty blood and sweat of normal labor and childbirth, allowing them to swoop in and save the day with sophisticated technological equipment and operations, and in the process reinforcing faith in the power of the medical establishment to "save" women from their own bodies.

The "Natural Childbirth" Model

A second model of childbirth has become increasingly visible in Israel over the past fifteen years. Unlike their mothers and grandmothers, most of the women of this study had either attended childbirth preparation courses, or read self-help or natural childbirth manuals. Prepared childbirth courses encourage the participation of fathers-to-be and the acquiring of information by the parents-to-be.

Childbirth preparation courses and books generally treat pregnancy as a matter over which women have a great deal of control through, for example, diet and exercise. Karen,[7] an American-born midwife, found in her experience that childbirth preparation class had a greater effect on women's behavior during labor than any demographic characteristic (for example, ethnicity, age, religious identification). Women who had not had preparation "freak out, their eyes go wild, they scream 'Mama,' they are tense, and less likely to bring their husbands with them." In the literature used in childbirth preparation courses, a key concept is control. Women are told that by learning about the childbirth process, about hospital routines, delivery options, and pain-reducing techniques they will feel more in control during birth. They will have better control over their own bodies (labor will proceed more as they would wish), better control over treatment (they will be calm and knowledgeable enough to ask for or refuse medication), and better control over their husbands (they will be able to tell their husbands how to help them during labor and delivery). In short, childbirth education offers women some sense of control and the result, according to Karen, is that they do not "get sick" during childbirth—they do not "freak out" or have "wild eyes." Even a six-week course gives women some measure of self-empowerment that translates into empirically better health.

Still, it is crucial to remember that the natural childbirth model is a foreign import—it is not Jewish, not Israeli, and not invented by Israeli women to express their own needs and demands. With its modern, American aura, it tends to be seen as a source of authority external to birthing Israeli women. In the discourse of the natural childbirth movement (at least as it is presented in many of the courses attended by pregnant women in Israel), birth is described as a test of personal achievement; the successful birther is one who avoids pain-killing medication and caesarian sections. In some of the courses, women pick up the message that medical interventions during birth represent a failure on the part of the woman, a message not very empowering for women giving birth in hospitals in which some measure of medical intervention is the norm. In my own study I found that while most women had some passing acquaintance with natural childbirth techniques (especially controlled breathing), most (not all) felt that the techniques were not particularly helpful: "I meant to use the breathing I learned in the course, but labor was too intense and I forgot to." Some of the women (mostly among those born in America) explained that they had chosen Misgav Ladach Hospital because they wanted a natural childbirth experience, but it turned out that a variety of medical interventions (induction of labor, caesarian sections, fetal monitors, episiotomies) were necessary in their specific case. Typically, women explained that, "My case was exceptional; the doctor said that he did the c-section just in the nick of time"; "In my case there was terrible danger"; or, "The doctors were wonderful, life-savers, the baby was in distress and they saved him."

Much of the natural childbirth movement, like many self-help and alternative medicine movements both in Israel and abroad, tends to privatize women's distress and thus disguises the social causes of illness and the cultural formation of "appropriate" medical treatment. Given a cultural context of belief in women's physical and especially reproductive vulnerability, natural childbirth teachings (especially in the somewhat diluted form typical of hospital-sponsored prenatal classes) may actually detract from women's sense of accomplishment at birth. I would even go so far as to suggest that the usually rather brief childbirth preparation courses offered to women who will give birth in highly medicalized and authoritarian settings (as almost all Israeli women do) tend to doom women to feeling that they have failed and that their failure represents a personal moral or physical deficiency, which was miraculously rectified by the doctor-savior.

Still, choosing natural childbirth must also be seen as constituting resistance to the medical model, in that it conceptualizes the birthing mother as potentially in control of her own body and capable of determining her own childbirth experience. That this conceptualization often fails to play out can be attributed to the tenacious hold of the state-supported medical establishment.

The Formal Jewish Model

A third model—the formal Jewish model—construes parenthood as an obligation for men (by the letter of Jewish law women are not obligated to bear children, but in practice men's obligation devolves upon women; "barrenness" is a legitimate reason for men to divorce their wives) and as a divine reward granted or withheld pursuant to proper behavior on the part of the human community. While children are welcomed and desired, childbirth is a source of *tum'ah* (pollution) for women, requiring purification rituals (in Biblical law the bringing of a sacrifice, in contemporary Jewish law immersion in the mikveh one week following the cessation of bleeding).

The control of reproductive resources (that is, women and children) via regulation of women's sexuality, allegiance, mobility, and agency is, of course, the bedrock of patriarchy. By means of myth and ritual, religion mystifies and camouflages these goals and sacralizes the processes by which they are attained. Most Israeli women have some contact with the formal Jewish model of childbirth. This may begin at the wedding, when brides routinely are blessed with the words with which the Biblical matriarch Rebecca was blessed: "May you be a mother of thousands of myriads," assigning, as Prime Minister David Ben Gurion well understood, national significance to women's childbearing. For Orthodox and ultra-Orthodox women, the formal religious model touches their lives if they bleed during pregnancy, in which case couples who observe laws of menstrual pollution refrain from physical contact because of the woman's impurity for a week after the bleeding ceases. Many traditional and almost all Orthodox and ultra-Orthodox couples refrain from touching once bleeding starts during the birth—a restraint that, with few exceptions, the women with whom I discussed this matter confided they find difficult. Several women volunteered that, "I don't think of myself as *t'me'ah* [polluted, in this case as a result of childbirth]," while others declared "I feel *t'me'ah* and how!" While the formal religious model has less direct impact upon the birthing experiences of secular women, it remains the case that eight days after the birth almost all Israeli women symbolically turn their newborn sons over to the world of men and the ritual circumciser, a ceremony many of the women whom I interviewed described as "very hard for the mother."

The "Folk" Religious Model

In addition to the formal Jewish rituals surrounding childbirth, almost all women with whom I spoke were familiar with traditional folk religious models of childbirth.[8] Israel is ethnically mixed, and rituals of the various ethnic groups have somewhat merged in popular culture (Zenner 1965). Shops in Jerusalem and other cities carry ritual accouterments such as pictures of famous rabbis and assortments of amulets. Even thoroughly secular pregnant women are repeatedly blessed by relatives, friends, and total strangers with the words: "It (the birth) should be in a good and auspicious hour." The folk model, like the formal Jewish model, stresses the need for divine protection; like the medical model, it emphasizes the dangers of birth.

Folk Religious Rituals

Rituals to Safeguard the Pregnancy

Carry string that has been wrapped around Rachel's Tomb
Seek many rabbis' blessings
Wear blue stone
Wear red stone
Avoid cemeteries
Send husband to holy tombs
Visit many tombs
Pray a lot
Make pilgrimage to holy tombs in Meron
Make pilgrimage to tomb of holy 'HaAri' (kabbalistic saint)
Seek blessing from one's own rabbi
Avoid eating radishes
Light Sabbath candles
Petition God while lighting candles
Make personal prayers occasionally
Make personal prayers constantly
Carry protective card
Visit specialist rabbi
Send letter to Lubavitch Rebbe
Wear red thread
Think about it during morning prayer
Send husband to talk to rabbi
Say special daily prayer
Give to charity daily
Visit grave of Baba Sali
Eat food blessed by special rabbi
Wear written amulet
Try to pray the formal service daily
Have husband say special prayer
Refrain from choosing name for baby
Bake Sabbath bread
Give money to synagogue after nightmare
Keep picture of Baba Sali in purse
Keep Book of Psalms in purse
Repair *mezuzot* (ritual objects) of house

Rituals Before or at the Birth to Ease Childbirth

Pray to God to help
Hold book of Psalms
Keep picture of Baba Sali
Place special stone in bra
Give to charity during pregnancy
Carry red thread from rabbi
Mother light candles at home
Recite psalms
Husband recite psalms
Husband pray
Phone rabbi for blessing from hospital
Recite *Sh'ma* prayer
Immerse in ritual bath in ninth month
Husband recite special blessing at synagogue in the ninth month
Eat ritual post-Sabbath meal
Husband learn Torah
Mother-in-law light candles
Husband open ark at synagogue
Bring Psalms to hospital
Bring *Book of Raziel* to hospital
Pray with husband and children
Give to charity when contractions start
Wear ribbon from saint-rabbi
Wear key from special rabbi
Say "*yehi ratson*" prayer
Eat apple on day of birth
Pray morning service on day of birth
Husband bring saint's cane to hospital
Light candles before a c-section
Keep amulet under pillow in hospital
Make personal petitions of God
Husband go to ritual bath
Go to Tomb of Patriarchs for special prayer on day of birth
Brother get blessing from famous rabbi
Pledge money to charity
Refrain from any ritual because it is forbidden for birthing woman to say the name of God
Uncle go to synagogue
Keep Baba Sali picture under pillow
Keep psalms under pillow
Husband say "Rabbi Hida'a prayer"
Purchase letter in Torah scroll
Recite *Shir HaMaalot* prayer
Husband get blessing from his own rabbi
Go to Western Wall night before scheduled c-section

Ritual Objects Placed in Newborn's Crib

Written amulet
Chapter from Book of Psalms

Salt under pillow
Picture of Rabbi Yosef Haim
Book of Psalms
Key
Book of Tania
Amulet from circumciser
Hamsa (hand) next to bed
Unknown book
"Everything"
Ribbon against evil eye
Shir HaMaalot psalm
Special amulet for before circumcision
Red ribbon
Pictures of rabbis
String
Book of Raziel
Kabbalistic written amulet
Candies

During our conversations, the women in my study talked about the folk rituals they had performed during pregnancy, birth, and immediately after the birth. As can be seen in the composite lists in the accompanying table 1, the folk rituals sort into three categories: to safeguard pregnancy, to facilitate birth, to safeguard the newborn.[9] These rituals are not required by Jewish law, although they do use Jewish symbols and concepts. I suspect that further field work would have doubled or even tripled the length of each list, and I suspect that if I were to repeat the study today I would discover that some of the rituals on the list have dropped out of the active Israeli ritual repertoire while many other rituals have been added. Even without careful attention to the content of the rituals, the sheer number indicates the extent to which Israeli women's childbearing experiences are ritualized.

Perhaps the most reiterated theme in the Israeli childbirth ritual repertoire is that of dependence: Myths, symbols, and rituals depict the vulnerable maternal female body as in need of expert help, whether from physicians, rabbis, or God Himself. Israeli women, like women around the world, tend to be physically and financially vulnerable during pregnancy. Pregnant women in Israel believe that hard work or intense physical activity will lead to miscarriage; pregnant women "need" their husbands to mop the floor and carry groceries. Employers may be reluctant to hire a visibly pregnant woman, further ensuring her financial dependence upon her husband. Pregnant women in Israel are inundated with the blessing that, "You should rise up alive from the childbirth bed," which encourages feelings of physical vulnerability and fears regarding who will take care of the children if the pregnant mother should die during birth. Folk religious childbirth rituals echo, and draw women into, the Jewish mythic corpus in which it is difficult to think of women who successfully managed, without "higher" intervention, to conceive, birth, and raise children.

Sh'mira *and the Interpenetration of Childbirth Models*

The various childbirth models that I have outlined interpenetrate in the experiences of individual women. Both the folk model and the biomedical model surround pregnant and birthing women with rituals that remind them that control does not lie in their own hands. The amulets, prayers, rabbis' blessings, and visits to holy tombs of the folk religious model are paralleled by medical rituals including sonograms during normal pregnancies, and shaving pubic hair, episiotomies, enemas, and fetal monitors during normal births. The folk model assimilates neatly both to the medical and the natural childbirth models: If God has decreed that there will be problems, neither modern medicine nor self-help will be of any use. For many women, the role of religious rituals is to beg God to grant that secular rituals and modern medicine will work.

The Hebrew word *sh'mira*, used by many of the women of this study, highlights the merging of the various models. Literally meaning "guarding," *sh'mira* (short for *sh'mirat herayon* or "pregnancy protection") refers to the bed rest frequently prescribed by Israeli doctors to avert miscarriage and "guard" the pregnancy (despite little evidence that bedrest during the first trimester has any effect on the likelihood of miscarriage [Pritchard and MacDonald 1980, 594]). When women are "on *sh'mira*," the implication is that doctors are actively guarding vulnerable female bodies, and that women (by remaining more or less immobile) are passively guarding their fetuses.

The word *sh'mira* is also widely used in Israel to mean protective rituals, prayers, or amulets. Many pregnant women engage in both kinds of *sh'mira*—women would describe themselves as "on *sh'mira*" for part of the pregnancy, and as having "worn it [an amulet] for *sh'mira*." *Sh'mira* in the latter sense has to do with God's guarding vulnerable pregnant women and babies (a popular appellation for God is *Shomer Yisrael*, Guardian of Israel). The implication of folk religious *sh'mira* is that the evil eye (either in the sense of vague harmful forces or in a more specific sense of ill luck wished on one by a jealous acquaintance) needs to be guarded against, and that women need help to carry out the task.

An equally common meaning of *sh'mira* in Israeli culture is the ubiquitous guard duty performed by soldiers. Pregnant Israeli women have husbands, brothers, fathers, and sons who do, did, or will do military *sh'mira*. Everpresent *sh'mira* by soldiers (and by hired guards in malls, movie theaters, and so on) reflects the national sense of vulnerability to enemy attack. Unlike the bedrest and amultets *sh'mira* of pregnant women, soldiers' *sh'mira* involves the ultimate symbol of personal empowerment: a large and visible assault rifle. These overlapping meanings of *sh'mira* strengthen cultural notions of men's soldiering and women's birthing representing parallel, yet fundamentally unequal, contributions to the collective. Men "do" *sh'mira*, women are "on" *sh'mira*.

The Stories Women Tell

A Heavy Burden to Bear

When I interviewed her, Rivka was thirty-eight, a secular, Ashkenazi, Israeli-born woman. Being a social worker was a significant part of her identity, but in the hospital context in which I interviewed her, other identities prevailed: specifically, her identity as a post–caesarian section patient. Rivka had wanted a natural childbirth and that is why she chose Misgav Ladach Hospital in what turned out to be a fruitless attempt to exercise authority over her body and childbearing experiences. When she arrived at the hospital the doctors decided to induce labor. After several days at the hospital, the doctors decided that the induction was not working. "The doctors tried to threaten me into a c-section. They told me that the baby may be born retarded if I don't do it. This made me so angry. Finally, one midwife said to me, 'It seems that you are thinking more about the birth'—I understood that she meant thinking about myself—'than the baby.' This had a big impact on me and I decided to have the c-section."

Rivka's self-doubt was a dominant theme in her narrative. For instance, I asked her what if anything she had done to safeguard the pregnancy or the baby, a question that most women in the study easily answered with lists of rituals or "careful" behaviors. Rivka replied that she had done "Nothing. I was very naïve." Rivka's critique of her own fertility behavior continued through to the end of the interview, when I asked her if she had accepted gifts for the baby during the pregnancy (accepting gifts before the birth is believed by many Israelis to elicit the evil eye). Rivka replied that she did not accept gifts, but added in self-criticism, "Not accepting gifts—that's a superstition."

Rivka's story underscores the combination of responsibility without authority that characterizes the childbirth experiences of Israeli women. By reminding her of her "responsibility" to the baby, the midwife and doctors convinced her to accept a medical procedure that she did not want. She blamed herself for abnegating responsibility during the pregnancy ("I was very naive") and she had disdain for herself for following the "superstition" of not accepting baby gifts before the delivery. At the same time, she made it clear that in the final analysis she had little authority over what happened to her body.

Shira was thirty years old, ultra-Orthodox, and American-born. She made a point of immediately letting me know that she was "more religious" than her family and that her attitudes and behaviors during pregnancy and childbirth had been learned in Israel. She graduated from college but did not work outside the home. She had five other children, and throughout our conversation she expressed concern about them. "My thoughts are at home. One kid is sick." In addition to the six births, Shira had had two miscarriages, one before this birth and one after the third baby. All of her adult life had been spent pregnant, trying to become pregnant, recovering from a pregnancy, dealing with problem pregnancies, or recuperating from miscarriages.

During this pregnancy, she took vitamins, "but I was not so careful [to avoid strenuous activity] and so spotted in beginning." Shira held herself responsible for avoiding or causing miscarriages, when in fact she had five small children at home and could not possibly "take it easy"—she had no control over the extent of her housework responsibilities. The sense of responsibility without true authority emerged in her comments about amulets: "I wore a ruby next to my skin during the pregnancy as a charm not to miscarry. My husband told me to do this, he read it in a book [she doesn't know what book]. I didn't do it in the pregnancy in which I miscarried. I've done this since the first miscarriage, but forgot last time [the time she miscarried]."

Shira continued,

> This pregnancy was "interesting." Staining in the beginning. I was in bed two weeks with mononucleosis. It was stressful emotionally and physically. The ninth month was difficult, the baby was big. The doctors scared me; they told me that I had another virus besides mononucleosis and because of that virus I should have an abortion. I did not even consider it.

Shira remembered feeling fear during the pregnancy that, because of the mononucleosis and the virus, the baby would not be healthy. To overcome the fear, "I said to myself 'It's not in my hands. If it happens it's because it was meant to be.' Also I would pray." Shira emphasized that to safeguard the pregnancy and make the birth easier, she did what her husband found in books, "not old wives' tales."

We talked about the birth. Shira was well informed regarding childbirth options and was a firm and knowledgeable believer in natural childbirth. Still, somehow the birth process spiraled out of her control. "The water broke and so they induced labor, and so I had really hard contractions. [Induction of labor typically leads to more intense contractions.] Then I hemorrhaged. That is why I [still] feel so weak. I was half in shock and they had given me *tishtush* [literally "fuzzy," which in Israeli childbirth culture refers to Demarol] and so couldn't hold the baby."

Shira's story, while distinctively her own—told with her particular blend of humor and resignation—illustrates a number of themes that run the through the narratives of many other women as well. Much of her adult life had been involved in the project of fertility, she held herself responsible for whatever "goes wrong" yet felt that she really had no control over "what happens," and she was engaged in continual interactions with men more powerful than she.

The Normalization of Illness

Israel's maternal mortality rate is laudably low (5.2 per 100,000 live births; see Reiss 1998, 76), a tribute to the inexpensive and easily accessible prenatal clinics provided by the government and to the universal availability of free obstetrical care for even the most complicated births. Yet maternal mortality statistics do not give a complete picture of the health implications of high natality for women. World Health Organization criteria for maternal mortality count deaths up to only forty-two days post partum, thereby excluding many if not most instances of maternal depletion (caused by repeated pregnancies and by closely spaced pregnancies). Nor do World Health Organization criteria include other potentially fatal conditions that have a slower developmental pattern. Pregnancy increases the risk of diabetes, hypertension, heart disease, gallbladder disease, and postpartum depression (Hoffman 1995), illnesses that do not necessarily "kill" women immediately, especially in a country with a medical care system as sophisticated as Israel's, but that certainly take a serious toll on women's health—often leading to what I call the "normalization of illness" even among quite young women.

Meirav was twenty-five years old, born in Israel to Syrian parents. She was ultra-Orthodox and had fourteen years education. When we spoke a few days after the birth she told me that she has been worrying about her other child, a sixteen-month-old. Meirav had a miscarriage between her last birth (sixteen months before) and this pregnancy. "I got pregnant fast. I didn't want to get pregnant so soon. I was still so weak from the previous pregnancy." Meirav had had three pregnancies in two years, a heavy physical load for her body to carry, compounded by her feeling that she had no control over the timing of the pregnancies. "This pregnancy was hard. *I had a lot of pains. But it was a normal pregnancy*" (my emphasis). In Meirav's remarks I draw attention to the normalization of pain and powerlessness, conditions that for Meirav seem to loop back on one another: Feelings of powerlessness led her to accept pain and illness as normal conditions, while pain and illness left her too debilitated to question or resist authority.

Leah was twenty-two years old, born in Israel of Moroccan parents. She had had ten years of education, identified herself as religiously "traditional," and had two other children at home. During the pregnancy she carried a card for *sh'mira* (protection, blessing) of the childbearing woman and the baby; the card was given to her by a stranger. "This pregnancy was normal," Leah explained, "I throw up a lot in all my pregnancies." Several times during our conversation, Leah exclaimed that holding the baby and breastfeeding right after the birth were important to her; that was how she bonded with the baby. When the baby was born, "I cried from happiness, didn't know what I was doing . . . Then they stole her[10] and then brought her back."

Interwoven with her elation at the birth of her daughter, Leah told a tale of loss of control. At the hospital the baby was "stolen" from her; after the birth she "didn't know" what she was doing; during the pregnancy a total stranger gave her a protective card and she meekly accepted it; she "throws up a lot" in all of her pregnancies yet had not used any form of contraception and had taken no breaks between her pregnancies. In fact, she saw sickness (throwing up a lot) as an expected "normal" state: At the age of twenty-two, Leah had accepted illness as normal.

Danger and Fear

Despite some ethnic differences (for a fuller discussion, see Sered 1993), I am struck by the pan-Israeli character of most of the beliefs and practices described by the women; I have recorded informants' ethnic identities in this chapter primarily in order to make that character tangible to the reader. Almost all women engaged in at least a few rituals that are drawn from an extensive cultural menu, and rituals spread quickly, as attested to by American-born Nancy. At the time we spoke, Nancy was twenty-six years old. She had worked as a stockbroker on Wall Street before coming to Israel, where she married an Israeli man born to Moroccan and Turkish families. Nancy said that during the pregnancy and birth, "I had no fear for myself although Israeli women tried to instill it in me." And indeed, they were successful, at least in as much as Nancy's ritual package was no smaller than those of other informants. That the culture of powerlessness and fear spreads is illustrated by women such as Israeli-born Orna, who wore a red stone amulet "because a friend gave it to me and I felt spooky giving it back, but I really don't get into that stuff."

The folk culture of childbirth in Israel constructs pregnancy and childbirth as dangerous events. It is "forbidden" to tell a pregnant woman "*mazel tov*"—offering congratulations implies that she has already achieved something, when, according to the Israeli view of things, unnamed dangers (over which she has little or no control) still lie ahead. More than one informant told me that "I wasn't scared of giving birth, but when people told me that, and when they told me '*she-takumi be-shalom*' [may you rise up from childbirth healthy and whole], I began to be afraid." The aura of danger that surrounds childbirth is what leads even women who believe strongly in natural childbirth to accede to a wide variety of medical interventions, and what leads even thoroughly secular and skeptical women to accept amulets.

Many women are swept up by fears of dangers hinted at by their doctors. Without access to more or to alternative information, most pregnant women undergo a variety of prenatal tests, experience days or weeks of fear waiting for the results, and then are either diagnosed as "sick" and swept further into the treatment system, or told to return for another test next month, restarting the process of pre- and post-test anxiety. Having lived on the anxiety rollercoaster for nine months of pregnancy (and often for months of prepregnancy fertility "problems"), the birthing woman entering the hospital is ready to believe that her birth is dangerous, and that she must surrender fully to the authority of the midwives, doctors, and rabbis.

Liat, a twenty-six-year-old Israeli-born secretary, had planned a birth without medication. But like so many other women, she found herself pulled into the culture of illness. To begin with, it took eight months to conceive—in her words, "a long time." The result of her culturally construed "infertility" was that she entered the pregnancy and birth process already thinking of herself, and thought of by others, as "problematic." She explains, "The pregnancy was okay, though they thought the baby had not developed right. So I was on *sh'mira*. Then the baby was in the wrong position, so I had a c-section."

Deborah was twenty-nine years old, born in America, and married to a man whose family came from Algeria. She was an Orthodox Jew and a teacher. Deborah spoke candidly of how fertility problems led her to be drawn into a ritual world not of her own choosing. I spoke to her five days after a c-section, her second one. This c-section was unplanned, but vague "things" unfortunately "went wrong." Deborah reiterated that during the birth, "I did not feel in control, I felt passive." She had had two miscarriages ("many problems") and it took her five years to conceive this baby. During the years of her fertility problems she consulted two local rabbis, one Ashkenazi and one Sephardi, but "I do not even remember what the rabbis said." Her in-laws went to the holy man Baba Sali and another rabbi.

At home there was an amulet under the pad of the baby's changing table: "The circumciser put it there last time and I left it there." Deborah did not believe in "all kinds of rituals," but she did put a *hamsa* (hand-shaped amulet) on the diaper bag at home.

Rabbis and Other Holy Men

Zehava, thirty-six years old, was born in Israel of a Moroccan father and Tunisian mother, had had fourteen years education, and described her profession as "good mother." She embraced an ultra-Orthodox life as an adult, and made frequent references to God and other religious matters. Our conversation took place seven days after her c-section. Right away Zehava told me that, "It feels good to be a mother." This was her fifth c-section, following seven years of infertility. The number of years in which she had been involved with pregnancy, then, include the seven years of infertility, the five times nine months of pregnancy, the five times one month of recoveries from c-sections, plus an extended period after her second pregnancy in which she was very sick. In addition to the years in which she had been busy with the social role of mothering a houseful of infants and toddlers, there had been more than twelve years during which her attention (and the attention of neighbors, relatives, rabbis, and medical specialists) was directly focused on her maternal body.

Zehava was very ritually engaged during her pregnancies. She went to the Western Wall and to Rachel's Tomb to pray and she sent her husband to pray at other holy tombs because, she told me, "His prayer is more effective." Moreover, she explained, pregnant women should not go to tombs (except of saints) because there are souls that did not finish their path in life and want to come back, "and so when they see a pregnant woman they go into the baby, and then the baby will only live a few years." Zehava told me that her husband puts a book of psalms and a special prayer for newborn babies (*Sh'mira LeNolad*) in the baby's crib, but that she does not feel that this is important.

Throughout our conversation, Zehava made repeated references to her years of infertility—the memory had not faded despite giving birth to five children. "When I was infertile my friends treated me like an outcast, not to come near me. I wasn't invited to circumcisions and weddings, and if a pregnant woman or new baby was mentioned in front of me, everyone would start saying '*bli eyin ha-ra*' [an incantation to keep away the evil eye] over and over. It was as though they thought I ate babies."

This time she became pregnant when her doctor said she could. She felt a close connection with Dr. R., who took her as a private patient even though she didn't pay him. (The usual system in Israel is for birthing women to be attended by midwives and if necessary treated by the physician on duty; it is relatively rare—and expensive—to have a "private" doctor attend one's birth.) "After the baby is born I only care about the baby and me. Not my husband. It's as if I blame him." Right after the birth, "I thank God that I have come back to my children, and that I will raise them and not someone else. I tell my children that they are all that I have." Zehava felt no connection to the midwives who do most of the maternity work in the hospital. I asked her who was with her during the birth: "No one, only the doctor and God."

Zehava was somewhat atypical in describing such a long period of infertility. Many more women in this study described themselves as having been "infertile" or having had "trouble conceiving" when the length of "infertility" or "trouble conceiving" was between six months and one year. Although she was much younger than Zehava, Rachel's narrative included many of the same elements. Rachel was twenty-four years old, born in Iran, and married to a man born in Israel. She worked as a secretary and considered herself religiously traditional. This was her second child, a boy. The first, a girl, was six years old. Rachel had had two miscarriages, and it took one and a half years to conceive this time. "My doctor encouraged me." She repeated throughout the interview that she felt very close to her doctor.

During the pregnancy Rachel experienced intense dreams involving a variety of authority figures. In the beginning of the pregnancy, Rabbi Abuhatzeira (the Moroccan saint known as the Baba Sali) came and gave her a necklace and told her everything would be okay. Later on he came again and put his open hand on her hand and on her daughter's hand, "and took me for a walk in the fields." She also dreamed that yeshiva students would come to her and hug her and visit her house. During the pregnancy she carried out a large number of rituals to safeguard her baby. She went to the holy tombs in Meron, she tied a red string around Rachel's Tomb (a well-known ritual, the red string, after being wrapped seven times around the tomb, is worn as a charm for fertility, healing, or an easy birth), and she asked several rabbis for their blessings. One rabbi told her to get a certain kind of stone and to wear it next to her body. "He said that the stone must be red. My mother [she possibly meant mother-in-law] went to a store on Jaffa Road to get it. The man at the store sold her a brownish-blue one. He said this one is better. I always wear it in my bra. Like this, wrapped in paper so that the stone won't be right next to my body—it isn't permitted—it is a holy stone." She brought a book of psalms and a picture of the Baba Sali with her to the hospital to help her during labor and delivery, but she left them in her bag because she did not feel comfortable taking them out in the hospital. Rachel described the labor and delivery as "difficult, they didn't give me anything for the pain." I asked her if she felt in control: "Not at all! I did not have strength."

In Rachel's narrative I noted her many references to external sources of authority, and to her acceptance of their often incomprehensible behavior. Despite two miscarriages and (what most Israeli women consider to be) a longish period of infertility, she had no complaints about her doctor; indeed, she described him in superlative terms. A rabbi said she must wear a red stone during the pregnancy (he did not explain why red is special), and she sought out a red stone. A shopkeeper said a brownish-blue stone is better, so she wore a brownish-blue stone. Yeshiva students and holy men visited her in her dreams, behaving in bizarre ways, which she did not question—at least in her narrative. She brought ritual items with her to the hospital, but left them in her bag because the dominant hospital culture made her feel uncomfortable taking them out. Her labor was difficult and "they" did not give her anything for the pain, yet she seemingly accepted "their" judgment about the extent of her pain and her desire for medication. The one decision that she described making on her own and carrying through independently was the decision to wrap the stone in paper before putting it inside of her bra in order to protect or honor the stone, presumably from the polluting influence of her pregnant, female body.

Sarah was twenty-one years old, Ashkenazi, ultra-Orthodox, with thirteen years of education. She talked eagerly about her interactions with doctors and rabbis. "The midwives were nice. They related to me more than the doctors did. For the doctors, I am not important." Sarah continued, "When we got to the hospital to give birth we called the rabbi for a blessing . . . At the very end I wanted an epidural and called the rabbi to ask if it is okay. He said it is preferable not to but I can if I really need to. He said that the pains are 'love's travail' [*yisurei ahava*]."

Sarah was one of the few women to have noticed—or to have articulated in conversation with me—that "for the doctors, I am not important." Most women who had anything more than fleeting contact with a doctor praised the doctor's skills and patience, or, conversely, criticized the doctor for "scaring me." In either case, women reported a fairly expected pattern of hierarchical relationships, in which the doctor directed and controlled the childbirth experience. Sarah, in contrast, described feeling outside of the hierarchical loop of patients and doctors, and instead turned repeatedly to her rabbi not only for a blessing but also for medical advice—finding in the synagogue the figure of authority that other women found in the hospital.

The role of rabbis in Rachel's, Sarah's, and Zehava's fertility experiences merits comment. Tsippi, an ultra-Orthodox midwife, noted that among religious women, "If something goes wrong during the birth they go to the rabbi. If there isn't time to consult the rabbi, they get very upset. It's like they are talking to God when they talk to their rabbis." At the same time, Tsippi clearly understood the competing sources of authority that work in the system. She explained that most women are delivered by midwives (for which there is no cost at Israeli hospitals). Only about 10% choose to pay privately for doctors to attend their births. "Rich women and very Orthodox women want doctors. Especially American newly Orthodox women want doctors and quote their doctors like God. The doctor is the voice of authority for everyone."

Holy Books, Women's Bodies, and Cultural Narratives

Like many other Israeli women, Meirav (we heard part of her story earlier) tied her birth experience to wider cultural narratives. Meirav explained,

> At the beginning of the ninth month I dipped in the *mikveh*, this is a *t'vilah le-s'gulah* [an immersion as a charm]. This is a *s'gulah b'dukah* [a charm tested and proven to be effective]. On the day that I went into labor I ate an apple—because of Eve—to make labor easier.[11] I learned these things at home, my mother taught me and it is in a book we have at home.

Like many other informants, Meirav situated the source of authority outside herself—in the divine realm, in the anonymous "verifiers" of charms, in her mother, in unnamed "books" (written, needless to say, by holy men).

Meirav was not the only woman who, despite a significant education and full literacy skills, made ritual use of "some book, I don't know which one." Shuli, for example, a twenty-six-year-old, religiously traditional, Israeli-born woman put into the baby's crib "a book that my father-in-law gave. I don't know what the book is." Meirav, Shuli, Shira, and other women took it for granted that men were the only ones who knew what was written in the sacred books, just like doctors were the only ones who understood the Latin names of illnesses or who knew what the scrawl on the prescription pad meant. In both cases, a monopoly over valued knowledge becomes mystified through its inaccessibility to the "uninitiated" (in the Jewish case, women customarily were required to remain "uninitiated"—uneducated), thus reinforcing and legitimating social hierarchies. "Not knowing" what the book is, despite twelve or more years of schooling, is a ritual statement of disinterest, subordination, and powerlessness that reiterates traditional cultural narratives in which Torah learning allows men to transcend the profane world while women remain mired in corporeality.

Bodily Doubts

Constructing Infertility

Mary Douglas (1975; 1982) has helped anthropologists understand how physical bodies symbolically reproduce the anxieties of the social body. Israeli public discourse certainly blazons the collective anxiety that dwarfs all others—anxiety over national security and survival (see Arian, Talmud, and Hermann [1988] on the "religion of security"). Following Douglas, we perhaps can better comprehend why the women whom we have heard in this chapter describe fertility experiences circumscribed by bodily doubts—the fear that "something can go wrong," and the wholesale embracing of rituals and consulting of experts. Women's bodies bear the burden of the national mission of perpetuating the state, the state is seen as threatened and vulnerable, and women's bodies manifest feelings of peril and defenselessness.

Israeli women rarely are encouraged to space childbearing, and for many women involved in the race to conceive, any efforts to delay pregnancy may be understood as risking incurring the evil eye (which will then make it difficult to conceive later on) or simply as tempting fate. While no research has yet addressed the rate of self-perception of infertility among Israeli women, it is clear from reports in the media and from conversations with Israelis of all ages and most ethnic groups that many Israeli women consider themselves, or have at some point considered themselves, to suffer from fertility problems. The zealousness with which Israeli women embrace fertility treatments reflects government-mandated financing of the treatments, national promotion of motherhood as constituting "good citizenship" for women, and culturally constructed doubts that the female body can function well "naturally." This highly compelling constellation is infused with even greater power through its correspondence to a mythic tradition that presents female infertility as somewhat normative yet ultimately curable through "higher" interventions—a theme that echoes in the epigraphs concerning the Biblical matriarchs Sarah, Rebecca, Rachel, and Hannah with which I opened this and the preceding chapters.

While religious culture has played a major role in shaping attitudes toward infertility (and in shaping many of the traditional and nontraditional fertility rituals pursued by Israeli women), and while some of the current Israeli regulations concerning reproductive technology were developed with rabbinic input, infertility tends to be understood primarily as an illness, and thus for Israeli women almost always leads to intensive contact with the very powerful medical establishment. Medical treatment for infertility involves hormonal and surgical onslaughts on women's bodies, and is carried out by specialist physicians considered masters of almost mystically sophisticated medical technology. Women clients often become highly dependent upon these specialists, seeing them, I suppose, much as the Biblical matriarch Rachel saw Jacob, as able to give or withhold children.

Israel has the highest rate of in vitro fertilization usage in the world, and Israeli fertility specialists are global leaders (on IVF policy in Israel, see Shalev and Lev, forthcoming). Israeli law guarantees insurance coverage for IVF treatments at unsurpassed rates: Every citizen may receive as many as seven rounds of IVF up to the birth of two live children, as part of the basic basket of health services provided by Israel's government-supervised health plans. (In comparison, contraceptives are not part of the basic basket of services, although some health funds have begun to partially subsidize them.) Some clinics in Israel are known for not turning away any client, even those with the most minimal chances of bearing a child. That women flock to IVF is not surprising: If motherhood is a privilege and a duty, infertility is both pitiful and reprehensible. Israel's first Prime Minister, David Ben Gurion, made that clear when he equated men who evade military service with women who do not bear at least four healthy children.

Although Israeli discourse typically presents infertility as an objective and measurable illness, infertility is actually more of a cultural construct than a biological absolute. Forty-five-year-old premenopausal women who are happily raising three teenaged children are not seen as "infertile" even if they have not conceived for fifteen years. Nuns are not considered "infertile," nor are sexually active non-pregnant fifteen-year-old girls. In contrast, a woman who has carried a pregnancy to term yet delivered a stillborn baby or a baby who died in infancy might well be considered infertile. Susan Kahn interviewed ultra-Orthodox women for whom the pressure to bear many children is intense. One of her informants was receiving extensive IVF treatments including hormonal injections and surgery because she had been diagnosed with secondary infertility after the birth of her fifth child; everyone else in her neighborhood had at least eight children and she was desperate to keep up (1998, 19).

Infertility is the ultimate culturally created illness. With no necessary reference to discrete physiological indicators, certain women are diagnosed as infertile and treated by the medical establishment, often with hormonal drugs and intrusive procedures that may themselves generate infirmity, pain, and disability. According to the National Registry of the Israeli Association for Fertility Research, 23% of women who had become pregnant through IVF treatments in 1992 were hospitalized due to pregnancy complications, and almost half (47%) of the IVF births were by caesarian section (cited in Ifrah 1999, 44). Pat Spallone (1994) has overviewed the medical literature documenting the short- and long-term risks from the fertility drugs and hormones routinely used in IVF. Among the best documented health risks are high rates of miscarriage, ovarian cysts, damage to the ovaries, hyperstimulation of the ovaries (in order to extract multiple eggs), and multiple pregnancies (which contribute to higher rates of complications of pregnancies, preterm deliveries, and perinatal mortality).[12] This is in addition to the depression and stress that ensue when women enter IVF programs with high hopes of bringing home a baby, only to find that the real success rates are very low, and to the mood swings and general discomfort associated with the treatment itself.[13]

In a 1986 survey of Israeli IVF clinics, Alison Solomon found that nearly every clinic viewed male infertility as an indication for IVF. Moreover, male infertility was almost always framed in terms of deficient or defective sperm, not in terms of deficiencies or defects in the men who produce (or do not produce) the sperm. Men rarely undergo invasive or uncomfortable treatment for infertility; they merely produce sperm by masturbating, the sperm is improved in a laboratory, whereas "perfectly healthy women are expected to undergo dangerous, invasive and damaging hormone treatments, followed by surgery in order to have the sperm introduced into their bodies" (1991, 104–105). Thus while women who do not conceive are considered "sick" and made sicker by infertility treatment, infertile men are considered to be essentially healthy individuals who happen to produce defective sperm. They are neither construed as sick nor are they made sick by the treatment process.[14]

Breastfeeding

> These are the labors which a wife does for her husband: she grinds, and she bakes, and she launders; she cooks and she nurses her son; she arranges the bed and she works in wool.
>
> —Mishnah K'tubot 5:5[15]

While exact statistics on breastfeeding rates are hard to come by, there is good evidence that the typical Israeli pattern is to "fail" at breastfeeding. As we shall see, women tend to doubt that they will "succeed" at breastfeeding. These doubts receive heavy institutional reinforcement through the government-sponsored well-baby clinic ritual of incessantly weighing the baby and recording each gram of weight loss or gain (breastfed babies are self-regulating—eating as much as they need rather than sucking down standard amounts of formula, thus this ritual tends to send nursing mothers into a panic) and through the many attractive photographs of invariably smiling babies displayed on advertisements for infant formula.

When I asked post-partum women in the Misgav Ladach Hospital study whether they were planning to breastfeed their babies, the overwhelming majority of women gave answers along the lines of "If I'll have [milk]" or "If I'll have enough [milk]."[16] In an additional set of interviews conducted in 1999 with first-time Israeli mothers,[17] a related concern raised repeatedly was the belief (typically passed onto women during pregnancy) that breastfeeding can harm women's health in the short term through painful nipples and in the long run by depleting the mother's strength. In a 1995–1996 study, most—64% of the women who breastfed for longer than one week and then stopped said that their reason for stopping was "not enough milk"; 39% said that the baby cried a great deal; 26% said the baby was not gaining enough weight; and 31% of the women said they stopped breastfeeding because they returned to work (cited in Ifrah 1999, 45).

What scholars call "insufficient milk syndrome" is characteristic of rapidly developing societies in which young mothers no longer have access to the accumulated maternal knowledge of village midwives and grandmothers, but do not yet have access to modern books and educational tools that could provide guidance in breastfeeding techniques. The absence of lactation information is compounded by the nature of work in developing societies: Unlike in traditional villages, there is no mechanism for new mothers to rest and gradually build up their milk supply. Mostly domestic workers and factory workers, young mothers in much of the urbanizing Third World may be expected to return to work a day or two after childbirth (Van Esterik 1988).

Although many Israeli women say that they have insufficient milk, the rest of the "insufficient milk syndrome" scenario does not fit the Israeli case. It is true that Israeli physicians are not likely to impart much lactation information and few hospitals employ lactation counselors, yet childrearing in Israel is far from the lonely chore that is characteristic of newly urban societies. Mothers, grandmothers, mothers-in-law, and older sisters surround Israeli new mothers; a great deal of childbirth and parenting literature exists in highly accessible formats in Hebrew; it is not uncommon for post-partum women to be offered subscriptions to parenting magazines while they are still in the hospital; and while some well-baby clinic nurses are poorly informed regarding lactation, many others are well informed. Moreover, Israeli new mothers benefit from unusually liberal maternity leave rights—women continue to receive their salaries for twelve weeks post partum, and their jobs are held for them for one year. In many ways, the external factors influencing lactation success seem to be in place.

My suspicion is that many of the women with whom I spoke were giving voice to the ambiguities inherent in the heavy responsibility that they feel for their baby's growth and happiness (note that a common reason for believing that they do not have enough milk is that the baby cries "too much") in a context in which they feel little control or authority. Despite reading or hearing that milk supplies in healthy women increase and decrease in response to the baby's demand, Israeli women are well prepared to believe that their babies are hungry, that their own bodies cannot provide enough for their babies. This belief is nurtured both by grandmothers and by physicians. A frequent player in lactation scenarios is a grandmother who "feels pity [*rachmanut*]" for a crying baby, and suggests to the mother to "try to give him a little formula, just so he won't be so hungry." The "pity" felt by the grandmother is, in many situations, magnified, mystified, and mythologized by the grandmother's horrific experiences during the Holocaust or during the years of food shortages in the 1940s and 1950s. The grandmothers of the 1990s, almost all of whom themselves gave birth in the medicalized environment of Israeli hospitals, tend to be eager advocates of Western medicine.

Despite the heavy weight of cultural history and the grandmother's "pity," the young mother may have heard that offering a baby supplements can spell the end of lactation (because the baby sucks with less effort from the bottle than from a breast), and so she consults a physician. Typically, Israeli physicians know little about lactation, yet have few compunctions about giving advice. Women are told—and it sounds very logical indeed—that babies have a natural self-regulating mechanism; they only eat as much as they need. Therefore, there is "no harm" in offering the baby formula—he will only drink if he is indeed hungry. What this advice leaves out is that offers of formula may be welcomed even by well-fed little babies who are hardwired to love to suck. Once introduced to the easy flow of bottle milk, babies may no longer nurse enough to stimulate an adequate supply of breast milk, and the mother comes to see her own body as inadequate.

During the 1990s the Israeli Ministry of Health began a campaign to encourage women to breastfeed. For example, the Ministry put out (or sponsored, it is not clear from the credits) a special breastfeeding issue of the magazine *To Be a Family* (no date). The lead article, entitled "There Is Nothing Like Mother," presented an interview with Dr. Dorit Nitsan-Kloski, the director of the Nutrition Department of the Ministry of Health. Nitsan-Kloski had conducted research on Israeli patterns of breastfeeding in which she found, as I did, that between 50% and 80% of mothers in Israel begin to nurse, but after one or two breastfeedings, they stop. At the end of three months, only about 15% are still nursing.

In her role as nutrition director for the Health Ministry, Nitsan-Kloski has made it her campaign to teach women that it is important to give only breast milk until the baby is six months old. Yet in a typical institutional battle over women's bodies, her expert advice falls on the ears of women who by law are entitled to only twelve weeks paid maternity leave, not six months. And in case her very persuasive arguments in favor of breastfeeding might have discouraged some women from going back to work after the twelve paid weeks, the ministry's glossy magazine, replete with page after page of enticing advertisements for baby products—a tribute to the commodification of infancy—provides its own counter-tug at the maternal heartstring. Is the "good mother" a lactating body or a consumer body? Not even the Ministry of Health knows for sure.

Although the Ministry's breastfeeding campaign has not had much success and few Israeli women breastfeed beyond the earliest postpartum days, some members of the medical establishment are zealous in their critique of those stubborn women who insist on breastfeeding even when it is against the "best interests" of the child. On February 2, 1999, the newspaper *Ha-Aretz* ran a large article with the headline: "More than the Child Wants to Nurse: Nursing has Turned into a Litmus Test of Motherhood, Femininity, and Feminist Commitment. In this Situation, It is More Difficult to Recognize Breastfeeding Problems—Even if the Situation Causes Suffering to the Baby, And Even if it Endangers His Health." The article quotes medical "experts" who say that in the wake of encouragement for breastfeeding in the past decade, "there has been an increase in the number of nursing babies who need to be hospitalized because of dehydration." Professor Paul Merlov, director of the pediatric unit at Rabin Hospital in Petach Tikvah, explains that, "It can reach a situation that is truly critical. There is a rise in the concentrations of salts in the body, and babies arrive at hospitals in a state of convulsions and spasms." In the same article, another important doctor talks about women who insist on exclusively breastfeeding even if the baby does not gain weight. "It is a small number of women, but sometimes we have to make an effort to convince them to give a formula supplement. In those situations we show them the weight charts, and try to convince them by using objective statistics." The maternal body constructed in these remarks is one that can potentially kill her own baby without the "objective statistics" of the expert physicians.[18]

The new mother, caught in the vise of culturally esteemed authority figures, learns that she has no control over her own body's ability to work well and nurture a baby, and that she had better "accept her responsibility" and "stop thinking so much of herself," exhortations that may already be familiar to women who tried to resist the induction of labor, fetal monitors, or c-sections—or, alternatively, who asked for pain medication when the midwife or doctor deemed it unnecessary. In the context of Israel's fertility culture, a variety of authority figures typically treat women as having no needs that are not identical to the needs of their children, and occasionally treat women as if they actually are dangerous to their own children.

My informants' feelings that they may not (or are likely not to) have enough milk is one aspect of a fairly ubiquitous and deep distrust of women's bodies. We have seen that many of them were swept up into all kinds of medical procedures even though they had planned for a natural childbirth; when push came to shove, they were not able to trust their own bodies' and ideologies. Despite very low rates of infant mortality in Israel, the largely well-educated women of this study did not have faith in their bodies' ability to "rise up healthy and whole" from childbirth. Israel's infant mortality rates are among the lowest in the world (8.8 per 100,000 live births; cf. Reiss 1998, 27) yet the vast majority of the post-partum women with whom I spoke did not purchase or accept gifts of clothes or other equipment for the baby before the birth. The reasons that they offered included "It's psychological, what if I come home without a baby?"; "the evil eye"; "superstition"; and "that is our custom." Similarly, although Israel has a low maternal mortality rate (5.2 per 100,000 live births; Reiss 1998, 76), very few women brought clothes to the hospital to wear for the trip home. Most of the reasons offered for this practice sounded a bit hollow (at least to my ears): "My bag was already full"; "No logical reason *to* bring the clothes"; "I did not know what to bring"; "Why carry stuff, it will get wrinkled"; "Clothes were not on the original list of things to bring that I received at my first childbirth preparation course [three children earlier]." Two women articulated their self-doubt: "I did not know what would be. When it all ends fine I will tell my husband what to bring for me and the baby"; "I don't know what will be after [entering the hospital]." My sense is that few women were consciously frightened of dying in childbirth, but they did not quite trust their bodies to give birth successfully, produce a (healthy) baby, and return home fit enough to wear street clothes.

Breastfeeding, like infertility, pregnancy, and childbirth, is not an unmitigated "natural" event. Particular cultural conceptualizations of the female body, of the breast, of the mother-infant relationship, of food, and of hunger all construct the breastfeeding experience. The absence of day care centers at most workplaces in Israel means that while maternity is glorified, the basic services that would allow women to earn a living *and* to breastfeed their babies do not exist. Maternity is noble, but not in public places. Jerusalem City councilwoman Anat Hoffman was heaped with abuse and ordered to leave the council chambers when she breastfed her infant during a meeting. Even at one of the most liberal and determinedly egalitarian synagogues in Jerusalem, breastfeeding during religious services precipitated heated arguments that revealed the extent to which gendered corporeal conceptualizations underpin hierarchical stances in Jewish and Israeli culture.

Chapter 3

The Militarized Body

Rape and the Woman Soldier

Living in a militarized state places significant demands and imprints upon women's and men's bodies. "War societies"[1] such as Israel are characterized by the normalization of violence, the ubiquitous presence of weapons (almost always in the hands of men), and unquestioned conceptualizations of women as victims or potential victims. Galia Golan argues that countries in a state of war value the male child above the female, seeing in the male a potential brave warrior who may be called upon to make the ultimate sacrifice on behalf of his country (1997, 583). In Israeli society, military service is "equated with service to the Jewish collective and, as such, is constructed to be the basis for entitlement to full citizenship in the Jewish state, and in a sense . . . even for consideration as a normal human being" (Izraeli 1997, 133).

The veneration and inculcation of militarism may cultivate positive self-worth of sorts in boys and men, along with traits such as aggressiveness and "toughness" that have both positive and negative corporeal consequences for men. For women, the cult of militarism has few, if any, corporeal benefits. Israel's popular discourse of gender polarity construed in physical terms (that the essential difference between men and women is seen as bodily), coupled with the central and normative role of the male-warrior-citizen, problematizes the female body. How does society frame and interpret a body that does not fit the cultural prototype of combatant?

We shall see in this chapter that women's bodies are constructed and defined in relationship to the male warrior body. If the prototypical male warrior—the "muscle Jew" (see Boyarin 1997, 76 ff.)—is strong, hard, and healthy, women are weak, soft, and ill.[2] If the prototypical male warrior is invulnerable, women's bodies are penetrable and permeable—symbolically and actually rape-able. If the prototypical male body defends his state, women's bodies need to be defended. If the prototypical male body fights, women's bodies are fought over. If men are agents of the state, women are its symbols, representing the collectivity at its most vulnerable. If the prototypical male body is solid and reliable—standing ready to protect the collective—then women's bodies are erratic and undependable—defenseless and exposed. If the male body is dedicated to the lofty goals of the collectivity, women's bodies are mired in private projects of sexuality and motherhood. If the militarized male body is unafraid (see Levy-Schreiber 1998, 147 ff.), the militarized female body is prostrated with grief over a fallen son, or frantic with worry expecting the worst. If the prototypical male body is aggressive, women are victims or potential victims of aggression—a social identity that links women to the six million Holocaust victims who, in Israeli popular culture, are often described as "going like sheep to the slaughter" (unlike the new Israeli soldiers who, it is said, would most certainly have fought back). Within the parameters of this cultural logic, women—like other victims—are partially culpable for their own victimhood; the "better" path is that of soldiering.[3]

Dafna Izraeli points out that one of the acknowledged functions served by women in the Israel Defense Forces is "being constructed as the opposite of men" (1997, 152); women are the mirror image through which "true" (male) soldiering can be constructed. Military mobilization of men depends upon women playing the "proper" roles of being feminine; that is, prone to capture and worth defending (Sharoni 1994, 125). In Israel, like in many other societies, women's bodies are imbued with a heavy load of symbolism. Nira Yuval-Davis has suggested that, "As the biological 'producers' of children/people . . . [and] therefore, [literally the] 'bearers of the collective'" (1997, 26), women tend to be "constructed as the symbolic bearers of the collectivity's identity and honor, both personally and collectively" (45). Women typically are presented as the raison d'être of going to war, while being excluded from the collective "we" of the body politic, thus holding an object rather than subject position in the collective (47). What Yuval-Davis is describing is a particular sort of corporeal construction in which women's bodies carry the weight of national purity and honor, yet possess neither the power nor the strength to defend or define the nation. In contrast, men's bodies are culturally construed as the embodiment of agency and action. In Israel, where the IDF is supposedly a "citizens' army" and where the army ethos (at least in myth) proclaims that each soldier is important and that individual initiative is rewarded, the army can be understood as an ironically health-enhancing site of agency for men.

Even a cursory reading of Israeli newspapers exposes the national belief that the Israeli collectivity is vulnerable (to invasion and to world opinion)—constantly endangered and under attack. Pushing this thought a bit further, it seems to me that women's bodies "act" in a manner consistent with this cultural construction. Jean Lipman-Blumen (1984) has argued that patriarchal systems entice women to go along with their own subordination by convincing them that the system has everyone's interests at heart and that men are more competent than women to protect those interests. It is certainly the case that Israeli women accept and embrace men's protection.

The line between military and civilian life in Israel is relatively porous. This has implications for all citizens. The government is to a large extent dominated by former military men. Generals in Israeli politics include Yitzhak Rabin, Moshe Dayan, Arik Sharon, Yigael Yadin, Yigael Allon, Ezer Weizman, Chaim Herzog, Rafael Eitan, Avigdor Kalahani, Yitzhak Mordechai, Amnon Lipkin-Shahak, and Ehud Barak. Mayors of Haifa, Tel Aviv, Ramat Gan, Beersheba, and other cities have held high military rank, as have the CEOs of many public and private companies. While the power accumulated in the IDF seems to translate rather easily into civilian power for men, the same does not seem to be the case for women. When Brigadier General (Res.) Yehudit Ben-Natan, former head of the IDF Women's Corps, ran in the Labor Party primary elections in February 1999, she found that she received less coverage than other high-ranking retired officers entering the political world. "Politics is no less chauvinist than the military. [Male] generals who leave the army are the focus of incredible public attention. But I am the highest ranking woman officer to run for election and the public recognition I have received is very, very low" (*Jerusalem Post*, February 16, 1999). It seems that the fine line between the military and other spheres of Israeli life is as gendered as the institutions on either side of that line.

This chapter looks at two kinds of militarized female bodies: mothers of soldiers and women soldiers. As we shall see, both of these roles hold great iconic value in Israeli culture, a kind of value that translates into enormous national responsibility, yet little actual authority.

The Grieving Maternal Body

After the sacrifice [of Isaac] on Mount Moriah, Abraham returned to Beer Sheba, the scene of so many of his joys. Isaac was carried to Paradise by angels, and there he sojourned for three years. Thus Abraham returned home alone, and when Sarah beheld him she exclaimed, "Satan spoke truth when he said that Isaac was sacrificed," and so grieved was her soul that it fled from her body."

—Traditional midrash, from Louis Ginzberg, *The Legends of the Jews*

> I feel these things, I live with these fears. The day my firstborn went up to Lebanon was the day I had to start going to a hairdresser to dye my hair. All of a sudden, I became an old woman. And you think about death all the time. —SMADAR BAR-ADAM, mother of two paratrooper sons, in *Jerusalem Post*, June 6, 1997

> And I will finish in a song of praise [*hallel*], praise to the Jewish mother, to the Israeli woman, who worries day and night, the woman who takes care of her home, of our children, the woman who is an integral part of our personal and national life, whom we could not do without. —PRIME MINISTER YITZHAK RABIN in a Knesset speech honoring International Women's Day of 1993

Rivka Bar-Yosef and Dorit Padan-Eisenstark have argued that, "The pattern of mobilization [in the Yom Kippur War] immediately determined the division of the population into two sharply defined groups—the active men and the passive women and children" (1977, 135). Women were not involved in roles that contributed to solving the crisis. During the war,

> Sex images became more stereotyped, more polarized, and more complementary. The mass media . . . played an important role in creating, transmitting, and reinforcing these stereotypes. The trend was to present men and women in consistent images characterized by a few basic attributes: the masculine attributes focused upon the instrumental combat roles and the feminine ones on the supporting expressive roles . . . Not even the Prime Minister, Golda Meir, could evade the stereotyping, in spite of the rather masculine role of the Supreme Commander of a fighting army. Though her toughness was never doubted, she often appeared before the public as the grieving and loving Jewish Mother. (1977, 137–138)

The image of the weeping mother, as we saw in the epigraphs with which I opened chapter 1, is deeply rooted in Jewish culture. The archetypal Mother Rachel crying for her children adds cosmic and collective significance to the grief of each mother who mourns her soldier-son; Rachel's mythic image draws contemporary women into eternal reiterations of women's powerless tears shed in the wake of wars over which they have little control. Funerals of Israeli soldiers, often broadcast on television, have become political displays as top government officials "are shown comforting weeping mothers and commending them for raising up sons who were ready to sacrifice their lives for their homeland" (Sharoni 1994, 130). Rela Mazali interprets women's crying for, or over, their soldier-sons as a ritual role that reinforces the rite of initiation of male warriors. "The women supply a legitimate agreed-upon vehicle for the expression of fear, emotional relief. If they cry, they intensify the full and difficult truth of the rite and supply it with an important part of its significance. [And contrary to appearances] their tears and cries of protest do not challenge this ritual but rather are integral to it" (cited in Izraeli 1997, 136–137).

Anecdotal evidence suggests that many Israeli women literally become ill from their sons' military service.[4] The director of a hotline for parents of soldiers reports that the line has been inundated with calls, mostly from mothers, "calling with panic attacks.[5] Knocking knees, heart palpitations, insomnia. They complain that every phone call sends them into a panic because they think it's 'the' call" (*Jerusalem Post*, February 21, 1997). Mothers of soldiers report feeling worried and powerless to protect their children. "Two of my children are in the IDF. My adjustment as a mother, at least in the early stage of their being in the IDF, was very difficult—I felt various physical pains and sleeplessness . . . I see myself as a woman frightened and scared about what happens to my children and husband" (Shemer 1992, 440). Another woman explains,

> The drafting of my children was filled with many fears and much sleeplessness. They all served in elite units. Two in Lebanon during the war, and if I am still sane, it is a miracle. Right now my daughter is a soldier and my youngest son will be drafted in two weeks, and he also wants to go into the Paratroopers, and again will start my via dolorosa [*masa ha-yisurim*]. (441)[6]

Presentations in the Israeli media differentiate between fathers' and mothers' reactions to their children's military service. Fathers typically are shown to be proud of their children, especially those in high-risk combat roles, while mothers are shown to be worried sick. To take just one example, in a *HaAretz* (March 8, 1999) interview with women serving in traditional male roles in the IDF, we read, "When my father goes into the shop in our village, people give him respect." Later on, we hear about mothers: "If I step on a mine, or if my brother does, my mother will hurt to the same extent." In the view of this soldier, appointment to a prestigious job in the IDF neutralized *her* gender status (neighbors were proud of her accomplishments as they would be of a young man appointed to a prestigious job), but did not neutralize her mother's gender. The young woman may have entered a role previously closed to women soldiers (still not a combat role, as we shall see), but her mother remains locked in her mythically glorified maternal pain.

In *Quarter Before Joining the Army*, a popular manual for young people soon to be drafted, an exemplary young man about to enter the IDF is portrayed as choosing between the Commandos and the Paratroopers—two branches of the IDF known for risk-taking. "And also Mother has something to say: She wants me in the PX, the legal offices, or as an MP [all safe jobs]" (Ettinger 1993, 10). Further on in the book a photograph shows a tearful mother clinging to her tall, smiling son. A poem associated with the photograph relates how the mother has been trying to pull strings through all kinds of personal connections in order to have her son taken care of in the IDF, but none of this can do any good because the army is outside of her sphere of influence. Allotted responsibility to raise healthy children, Israeli women are deprived of authority within an institution that has the power to determine whether those children ultimately will live or die.

The Woman Soldier

The active enlistment of women as soldiers in the IDF can be seen as a form of resistance to the passive, grieving maternal body. In conversations over the past fifteen years with university students who had recently finished military service, I repeatedly heard of the passion, patriotism, and eagerness to do their part with which young women enter the IDF.[7] Yet once inside the gates of the IDF, most women find that traditional gender formulations are amplified rather than transformed, and the woman soldier is simply a younger and sexier version of the weeping mother, sharing her weakness, her vulnerability, and her exclusion from the world of male decision-makers.

The manifest dominance and symbolic importance of the IDF in Israeli society give special, sometimes even magical power to the identities constructed within it. The IDF plays a principal role in establishing gender identities and gendered bodies in Israel. A classic example of what Goffman (1962) calls a "total institution," the IDF has an especially strong hold over its members. During the period of a young man's or woman's military service, IDF culture and gender rules predominate; there is no other cultural reality to serve as a check to military culture. The IDF has near total power to shape citizens' bodies at a point in the life cycle in which adult bodies are emerging from adolescence.[8] Israeli men—particularly those serving in combat positions—undergo an intense three-year period of military service and then annual monthly follow-ups in which they actively and consciously train to be effective agents of the state. The position of women in the IDF is less clear; women are state symbols rather than agents, and the construction of symbols tends to be indirect, implicit, and mystified (cf. Lincoln 1989).

Despite Israel's universal conscription, it is simpler and far more commonplace for Jewish women than for Jewish men to avoid military service: Approximately 35% of eligible young women opt out. Jerby (1996) cogently argues that the wholesale exemptions granted to women link Arabs, women, ultra-Orthodox men (exempt from service while studying in yeshivas, they have come to be seen as draft dodgers by much of the population), and unfit men in the public imagination: None can be ideal citizens. While practices vary from year to year, there are two primary reasons for which women are allowed to claim exemptions: that they are Orthodox, and that they are married or mothers (unofficially, proof of two or more abortions is also grounds for exemption; see Jerby 1996).[9] Exemption for these reasons suggests a fundamental cultural incompatibility between the religious, married, or fertile female body, and the soldier body. I suspect that the practice of releasing married women from the IDF is a sort of "gentlemen's agreement" that acknowledges that women cannot serve two masters—a husband and a commanding officer. Exempting Orthodox women similarly eliminates the possibility that a rabbi and a commanding officer will make conflicting demands upon their bodies. The exemption of mothers is perhaps the most salient in that it institutionalizes the gendering of national missions: combat for men and motherhood for women.

The National Service Law (*Hok HaSherut*) of 1952 closed to women three categories of professions in the IDF: combat positions, professions in which surrounding conditions are not suitable for female soldiers, and professions that demand physical strength. In 1987 the Knesset essentially eliminated the law authorizing the Chief of Joint Staff to make rules regarding women's service, thus removing the legal basis for excluding women from these positions. Yet IDF policy has not substantially changed. For the most part, women in the IDF are perceived as, and sometimes officially defined as, "increasing the fighting power of the IDF by filling administrative and professional positions, in order to release soldiers, men, for combat positions" (Jerby 1996, 72). Iris Jerby cites figures regarding women's work in the IDF in 1993: 39% of women soldiers engaged in clerical work (down from 70% in the early 1980s), 36% worked as instructors (a broad category including both military instruction and educational work with disadvantaged youth), only 0.4% worked in computers, and 1.2% worked as drivers (1996, 73).

The fact that women are drafted in Israel reflects the egalitarian values of some of the pre-state and early state leaders and movements, and the insistence of Israeli women that they, too, can build and protect their country. The draft of women suggests that Israeli women resist the notion that men are the ones who defend passive "womenandchildren" (Yuval-Davis's term). Yet from the earliest days of women's service in the IDF, they have been excluded from positions of prestige and power. In a typically Israeli way, one hand gives and the other takes away. Women are drafted into the IDF—proclaimed full and equal citizens of the state. Yet service in the IDF means intense socialization into highly gendered roles in the context of a persuasive and powerful total institution. These are the kinds of paradoxes that take a toll on Israeli women: the omnipresent vision of equality and respect coupled with repeated reminders of social inferiority. The ambiguity of gendered discourses in Israel has the additional effect of opening the door for constant scrutiny of women's bodies, an activity at which, as we shall see, the IDF seems to excel.

In January 2000, the Knesset passed a bill allowing women to volunteer for all categories of jobs within the IDF. Still, it should be emphasized that women's volunteering and men's conscription do not place women and men on equal footing. Moreover, as Dafna Izraeli pointed out, the law makes no reference to issues of promotion. "As long as there are no women in senior decision making positions, no matter how many women run 80 kilometers along with men the rules of the game, the culture, the definitions of equality and what women may/can/want to do will be defined by men. One woman at the rank of general (as promised by the IDF Chief of Joint Staff) will make little difference. I have witnessed how the token woman is silenced without anyone even having to tell her to be silent" (personal communication).

Corporeal Differences

In IDF discourse, gender difference tends to be presented as bodily, a discursive device that functions to naturalize gender and gender hierarchy. This is clear in comments like this one by Brigadier General Orit Adato, Chief Officer for Women in the IDF: "We are beginning to see the trends changing for women [in the IDF], most importantly in areas that require *cognitive abilities*, such as technological courses, and pilots' courses" (*Jerusalem Post*, June 26, 1998; my emphasis). In areas that require corporeal abilities—or, to be precise, that require certain culturally agreed upon corporeal conceptualizations—trends have not changed at all. As Brigadier General Amira Dotan, a former head of the Women's Corps explained: "We recognize that there are *physiological differences* between a man and a woman, and I do not want to blur those differences" (*Ba-Machaneh*, August 17, 1983, quoted in Barnoy 1997; my emphasis).

On Independence Day of 1999 an Israeli newspaper ran a series of interviews with three exceptional young women serving in traditional "male" jobs in the IDF (*Yedioth Aharonoth*, 7 *Yamim*, April 16, 1999). The rarity of women soldiers in jobs that use guns or sustained physical strength lent an aura of the exotic to their stories. The issue of women serving in male roles is symbolically charged in Israeli culture—a measure of women's worth in and to the IDF, making these interviews more than just human interest stories. Both the way that the newspaper presented the women, and the way that the women presented themselves to the newspaper's reporter, exemplify the corporeal core of gender discourse in the IDF. Alongside each interview the paper ran a photograph of the young woman dressed in full battle gear, holding or aiming a large weapon and looking strong and purposeful. In addition, each young woman was shown in a snapshot in attractive civilian clothing and looking slim and wistful, clarifying that no deep gender transformation had taken place; these soldiers still had feminine bodies.

Each of the three women told the reporter that in the course of her work she endured gender discrimination and continuous sexist and sexual wisecracks. At the same time, these three IDF "success stories" explained that they too share in the Israeli discourse of gendering physical difference. For example, after declaring that she does her job as well as any man, Dorit Gofer, one of the young women, continued: "There is a physical difference between men and women and there always will be, nothing can be done about it. If there is a heavy load that I have to lift, it is very difficult for me, and in contrast someone else [a male] hoists it up with one arm, and even helps me . . . [But] in terms of emotional fortitude, there is no difference." Sivan Rozenblum, another of the women soldiers, made the distinction between corporeal gender (immutable) and behavioral gender (not immutable) even clearer: "There are differences between the sexes, and I don't think that it is a problem to say so. You see it here a lot in terms of physical things, and I don't think it is shameful to say so. Emotional fortitude is a thing that is learned. I am sure that now I have more than I did, and even more than other men."

The third woman, Idit Atiya, discussed the stigma attached to a woman working in a traditional male job: "It's like they expect to see girls [in this role] like 'tom-boys.' That they will physically look like boys because it isn't feminine to lug cables, to lift heavy equipment, and not to shower for a week. That comes from the idea of how a woman should look, and so if you are a woman you can't do it, and if you succeed in doing it, it means you aren't a woman, something is 'screwed up' in your genes." Atiya's comments underscore the Israeli gender scheme: If a woman acts "like a man" she must have "screwed up genes"; that is, the underlying cause of her "male" behavior must be corporeal. Atiya continued, "I have a chauvinist view of things. I think that men and women are totally different and that each has what is special to his or her sex, and we don't need to try to blur the differences. It is a fact that men have more physical strength, their average and their record are higher."

According to Orna Sasson-Levy, who has carried out research among women who have served in traditional male jobs in the IDF, the women who make it in male roles feel scorn for the weak "average" women of the IDF. This scorn, as I see it expressed in the interviews that Sasson-Levy has recorded, often is communicated in corporeal terms. One of Sasson-Levy's informants recalled her fellow female recruits in basic training before she herself was selected for her more challenging job: "Seven hundred thousand girls . . . each one with [cosmetic] creams, stuff . . . disgusting . . . seven hundred thousand [bottles of] makeup. Pathetic . . . I felt like 'blah' . . . like one of seven hundred thousand tits."

Sasson-Levy found many of these women soldiers depicted themselves as having adopted male corporeal and linguistic mannerisms. One young woman who began her military service in an office in Tel Aviv remembered: "I was made-up super-duper, in a way that today I never am made-up. My uniforms were always neat, and I always wore jewelry, always rings and [nice] shoes and everything, to look as fashionable as possible in the uniform." Her clothing style at that time fit IDF gender stereotypes and the specific demands of her commanding officer. After an officers' training course she went to serve in a base in the Negev Desert where the style was to wear oversized uniforms and informal clothes. "There at some point I started to learn that you have to say [vulgar slang] words like *jeaffa* [filthy] and *kus emek* [your mother's cunt]." Significant in this particular woman's experiences is her revelation of the way in which adopting "male" clothing practices was part of a larger corporeal program that included "learning" speech mannerisms that degrade women's bodies.

One of Sasson-Levy's informants talked about how carrying a gun affects the bodies of the (relatively few) woman soldiers who are given them: "Haven't you noticed them in the street? They walk proud and straight, striding like they know where they are going. You won't see her carrying a gun and strolling, looking around, not sure of her situation . . . She wants to get somewhere." Implicit, of course, is the portrayal of the normative female body that is "not sure of her situation" and does not know where she wants to go.

Another woman described the feeling of carrying an M-16: "Like a sort of decoration, a decoration I loved to wear because it is not a feminine decoration. I mean there is something I loved in it, to go around with a symbol of status that is not earrings, that it's not an adornment that is supposed to make me pretty, but rather something that I am very proud to have achieved. It's not like baubles, it's like walking with a book in your hand, a very important book that everyone can see." She explained that carrying a gun has transformed her from being a symbol to being an agent. She is no longer an adorned body but rather an active body—guns and earrings are not equivalent "decorations."

Moreover, and this is an especially cogent comment, she made explicit the connection between guns and a "very important book that everyone can see you carrying." Within Jewish culture there is only one "very important book that everyone can see you carrying"—the Torah. Guns and Torah scrolls indeed have a great deal in common: Both confer socially recognized power and status upon the one who (legitimately) carries them, and both are customarily understood to belong to men. In traditional Jewish culture, women are not permitted to touch the Torah scroll;[10] in contemporary Israeli culture, women are not permitted in combat positions and women soldiers rarely carry guns. Both guns and Torah scrolls are cradled in the arms of male bodies; both guns and Torah scrolls define maleness in culturally persuasive ways; guns and Torah are parallel direct and symbolic means that have been used to obtain and enforce the subordination of women. Unlike the women in chapter 2 who ritually denied knowledge of the holy books that protect their babies, this exceptional woman soldier has claimed for herself a visible symbol of power.

Neat and Sexy

The discourse of the IDF offers very different corporeal projects for men and for women. Divergent gendering of male and female soldiers begins in the pre-draft phase, when advice directed to young men focuses on physical fitness, on preparing them to actively defend their nation. Advice directed to young women focuses on improving their outward appearance—girls are told that they "represent" the IDF and so need to look nice (Levy-Schreiber 1998, 201 ff). Books and pamphlets read by high school students initiate the process of socialization into IDF culture. Throughout this chapter I shall quote from a popular book of this genre, *Quarter Before Joining the Army*, by Amos Ettinger, a colorful volume filled with glossy photographs of soldiers and written in a folksy rhyming style. Copies of the book have been handed out by the city of Tel Aviv-Jaffa to young people entering the IDF (an endorsement from the mayor of Tel Aviv appears on the first page), giving the book a seal of officialdom.

Behind the Shine

The uniforms are polished and bright.

—Amos Ettinger, *Quarter Before Joining the Army*, facing a photograph of a smiling woman soldier

The uniform and appearance of women soldiers have served as topics of newspaper editorials and radio and television talk shows in Israel throughout the years. The Hebrew name for the Women's Corps is an acronym "CHEN" which also means "charm" or "grace." (The Women's Corps, unlike the Engineering Corps, Air Corps, or Tank Corps, has no functional role; women in the IDF are members of CHEN but are assigned to other divisions for their work. There is no analogous "Men's Corps.") As national symbols, IDF women are expected to be attractive. Female attractiveness in IDF culture is comprised of two overlapping components: neatness and sexuality.[11]

A great deal of the very short basic training of women soldiers drills them in neatness. They are instructed in hygiene, given strict rules regarding hair length and style, and repeatedly checked for an orderly appearance. One senses that the body project of women recruits focuses less on preparing them for military readiness than on preparing them to present a certain image. The preferred image is a body that is orderly, controlled (shirt tucked in, and so on), and pleasant.[12] Informants and friends tell me that one of the more "annoying" aspects of basic training for women is the incessant inspections for neatness in clothing and in the barracks.

Looking at pictorial representations of Israeli soldiers, Edna Levy-Schreiber found that,

> The imagery of the ideal soldier that floods the mainstream Israeli media almost daily is of moving bodies—bodies running, firing and sweating . . . Male soldiers are almost always depicted according to this action framework. But if he runs, she smiles. Female soldier bodies wink, pose and look good. Body stance, facial expression and props in hand . . . signal a passive body that is all appearance. Control and discipline do not build up women soldiers' strength and stamina but keep women's bodies slim, neat, and looking pretty . . . the female effort is to appear as a static object. (1998, 173–174)

Posed pictures of women soldiers appear frequently in the press. "These women are neatly dressed, well coiffed, often wearing makeup and almost always smiling" (182). In other words, they are groomed for the scrutiny of the Israeli public. Moreover, I would add, in photographs in Israeli newspapers, women soldiers are often portrayed under the ritual scrutiny of male officers at graduation ceremonies, military parades, and so on. To take just one example, an article reporting on the first group of women to complete a grueling training course for combat fighters in the Border Police opened in this way: "The women of the Border Police squad snapped to attention for their Corps Commander's review, and their grips tightened on M-16 rifles held tightly against crisp, new uniforms" (*Jerusalem Post*, June 7, 1996). We shall return to the issue of "double scrutiny" in a later chapter.

Eyal Ben-Ari (1998) has argued that a critical expectation for male soldiers is that they learn control: control over their emotions, over fatigue, over fear, and over pain. It seems to me that the female soldier body is also taught control, but of a different sort. The female body is understood to be the antithesis of the warrior's body; it is erratic and undependable, conceptualizations well rooted in traditional Jewish culture. These are traits that do not fit well with military culture. I suspect that the sometimes obsessive concern with the neatness of women soldiers is part of a program aimed at coping with, and overcoming, the perceived instability and unpredictability of women's bodies. Unlike the body projects of military training for men, which prepare them to fight effectively, neatness in women soldiers is an end in itself. The neat female body is a body that is under total institutional control.

Girls Girls

In every profession and job, in instruction and command, an unwritten law, but a given, is that during military service you will find a husband.

—*Quarter Before Joining the Army*

The *Jerusalem Post* of May 2, 1996, reported that women soldiers complained that they were being sent to various events where they were treated like "cheap bar hostesses." One of the precipitating incidents (see *Jerusalem Post* of January 29, 1996) had to do with the IDF ordering fifty women soldiers to visit a British aircraft carrier docked at Haifa Port. The visit had been defined as a study tour but no studying took place, and only women soldiers were included. Apparently, after a ten-minute tour they were put in a bar with dim lights, romantic music, and alcoholic drinks, and were expected to provide pleasant company for male soldiers. While this particular incident may have been an extreme one, women soldiers are routinely sent as escorts for VIPs, and are often put to use presenting gifts or flowers to important people. (Colonel Anat Rotem, deputy chief of the Women's Corp, recently issued an order banning this kind of use of women soldiers.)

In her work on pictorial representations of women soldiers, Edna Levy-Schreiber has observed that the IDF spokesman's office has a "history of directing photographers to photo opportunities of women soldiers in scantily-clad pseudo-porn poses" (1998, 213). According to Levy-Schreiber, in the context of the IDF, "[W]omen's sexuality is not much different from women's sensitivity or prettiness; all are resources that make men's difficult job of soldiering a little more pleasant. In media portrayals women's sexuality is in service to male soldiers. Women are not the active soldiers, but good-looking objects and sexual providers" (225). Journalist Ron Adalist calls the IDF "the largest matchmaking agency [*mo'adon shiduchim*] in the country" (*Ma'ariv, Sof Shavua'*, April 9, 1999). This attitude was best summed up in the infamous slogan coined by President Ezer Weizman (in his younger days): "The best [men] to pilot school and the best women to the pilots."[13] It is telling that women conscripts are given information regarding birth control; parallel information is not given to male conscripts. This practice suggests that the IDF sees sexuality as "women's business."

In an unusually (and perhaps unfortunately) candid remark, Colonel Gershon HaCohen, head of the Seventh Armored Division, told an audience of high school seniors that traditionally men are warriors and women are prostitutes, and that most of what women do in the IDF can be replaced by office machines. Public reaction was highly critical and exceptionally revealing of cultural attitudes. Knesset member Shlomo Beniziri condemned HaCohen's word choice but agreed that this indeed is what many people think. "It is common knowledge that new male recruits are called 'fresh beef' and females 'fresh mattresses'" (*Jerusalem Post*, February. 3, 1995; see also Izraeli 1997, 129, for a discussion of this incident). While I think that both HaCohen and Beniziri overstated the case, each for reasons of his own (Beniziri represents the ultra-Orthodox Shas party, which is opposed to drafting women at all; HaCohen is a career military man), they did put their fingers on several fundamental matters: popular analogies between men's combat and women's sexuality, the conscription of women's sexuality into the national military project, and the understanding that militarization threatens women's bodies via sexual violence and abuse.

Women in Combat Positions: Endangered and Dangerous

> And then Dina, the daughter of Leah, born to Jacob, went out to visit with the daughters of the land, and then Shehem son of Hamor the Levite Prince saw her and he took her and he lay with her and he abused her . . . And the two sons of Jacob, Shimon and Levy, the brothers of Dina, took each his sword and came to the unsuspecting city and killed all the males [after tricking them into agreeing to be circumcised]. . . And then Jacob said to Shimon and to Levy, "You made me infamous among the residents of this land, the Canaanites and the Perizites, and we are small in number and should they gang up against us and smite us, that will destroy me and my household." And they replied, "Would you have our sister made into a harlot?"
>
> —Genesis 34:1, 25, 30–31

Israeli arguments against allowing women to serve in combat positions are consistently corporeal, echoing normative conceptualizations of gender in terms of bodily difference in IDF and Israeli culture. The discursive repertoire includes the opinion that women are not physically strong enough, that their behavior or skills are erratic because of the menstrual cycle, and that it is not worth investing in training women because they become pregnant or marry and leave military service earlier than men (a situation institutionalized by shorter required service for women). Another claim that intermittently enters discussions of women in combat positions argues that if women soldiers train with men they will distract the men and enter into romantic relations detrimental to the group as a whole (see *HaAretz*, February 27, 1997; byline Avirama Golan). Brigadier General Regev, the Manpower Branch officer responsible for placement in the Israeli air force, summed it up in his remarks to the Knesset Committee on the Status of Women in the aftermath of the first woman graduating from the air force pilots' school: Every woman takes the place of a man; women don't have the stamina to be pilots; it interferes with childrearing; there is high burn-out and effort in training; and "I also think it's not natural for there to be female pilots. And it's a fact that there hasn't been one for many years" (*Jerusalem Post*, December 29, 1998).

The "unnaturalness" of women serving in combat units (a discourse that presupposes that combat is somehow "natural" for men) has been particularly promoted by President Ezer Weizman. During a visit to an IDF base, Weizman offered his commentary on the High Court ruling that opened the way for women to serve in combat roles (the Alice Miller case): "Just as you don't see girls running after the ball together with men in professional sports, there is no place for combatant women in combat units." According to an article in the *Jerusalem Post*, May 27, 1996, Weizman had previously told Alice Miller directly, "Listen, missy, have you ever seen a young man darn socks?"

In November 1993, Alice Miller, who had trained as a pilot in South Africa, asked the IDF to allow her take the pilots' aptitude test. She was refused on the grounds that women are not eligible for combat duty. Miller petitioned the High Court to set aside as unlawful discrimination the IDF's refusal to admit her to the course. The argument made to the court by the IDF was narrow in scope: Women serve for less time (until age thirty-eight, versus age fifty-four for men) and are released if pregnant, so it is not financially or operationally feasible to train a woman as a pilot. Also, a woman pilot who becomes pregnant would be grounded for at least six months (medical considerations disallow flying in the last six months of pregnancy) and then would require expensive retraining.

More interesting, to my mind, were unofficial responses by air force sources to the court's ruling in favor of Miller's petition. According to a high-ranking air force officer quoted in the press, the ruling did not deal with the main issue at stake—society's willingness to deploy women in combat. "The issue is not a woman being a pilot. I have no doubt women are quite capable and qualified, perhaps even Lt. Miller. The real issue is, what next. She says she wants to be a combat aviator. Assuming she graduates from the course, then the real dilemma arises, because we have traditionally refrained from using women in combat positions for various reasons" (*Jerusalem Post*, November 9, 1995). These "various reasons," although not spelled out, were understood by all Israelis.

In the wake of women petitioning the High Court to overrule their exclusion from the navy's training course, Officer in Command (OC) Navy Admiral Alex Tal clarified that,

I have no doubt that women can be accepted into and complete the naval course. But it is society which must give its opinion whether we, as a society, are prepared for women to serve beyond the borders, set out on ambushes, serve in outposts, and on coastal patrol craft, missile boats, and submarines in enemy waters, exposed to all the dangers that male fighters are exposed to. (*Jerusalem Post*, April 1, 1998)

Admiral Tal's comments echo what I suspect is the dominant sentiment in Israeli society—that there is something worse about exposing women to danger than exposing men. The question this sentiment raises is why: Are women worth more? It would seem not, since they are paid, on the average, only about two thirds of what men are paid. Are women, then, particularly vulnerable to danger?

Israeli folk belief has it that women in combat positions could be taken captive by the enemy, in which case they are likely to be raped and possibly impregnated by enemy sperm. Furthermore, if women were to be captured, the IDF would have to endanger male soldiers by sending them in after the women in order to save them.

The argument that women soldiers could be raped has been part of the conversation regarding women serving in combat positions in other Western countries as well as in Israel (during the Gulf War the issue was raised in the United States), yet not nearly to the same extent. In a comprehensive discussion presented by three different authors in Nancy Loring Goldman's (1982) anthology *Female Soldiers—Combatants or Noncombatants?: Historical and Contemporary Perspectives*, numerous objections to women serving as combatants in the U.S. military are itemized: Women might break down under torture and reveal secrets to the enemy, women do not have enough physical stamina, women could be shot, women are more emotional and afraid of pain, women are less cold-blooded and steel-nerved in moments of crisis, women are not killers, women lose training time during pregnancy, someone would have to take care of the children of women combatants, having women in a unit could damage men's self-esteem and group bonding, women are naturally less combative, an army with women soldiers would be perceived by the enemy as weaker, and even, how would women soldiers dispose of tampons or sanitary napkins in the trenches. In that entire seventy-five-page discussion not a single one of the three authors even raises the issue of rape. While Israel is not alone in fearing the rape of women combatants, the sustained conscription of women over a fifty-year period has blended with deeply rooted cultural myths to make the issue one of the fundamental shapers of Jewish Israeli female corporeality.

The fear that women soldiers will be raped by the enemy is firmly anchored in Israeli culture. During the first stage of the 1948 War for Independence, women participated actively. While most women served in auxiliary roles, such as signaler and nurse, some served in combat roles alongside of men; women soldiers were not confined to the bases and outposts, and they were present on the front lines. Yet, according to Niva Yuval-Davis, "even when it was admitted (as was very often the case) that the women were as good, the male soldiers and commanders worried that they would be captured and raped by the enemy." At a later stage of the war, as the IDF became more institutionalized and Israel's position improved, "Instructions were given by headquarters to take women away from the front line (which still did not mean complete safety because of the small size of the country, but did decrease the chance of the women being captured alive by the enemy)" (1985, 658). Still today, according to Orna Sasson-Levy, "The fear that women soldiers will be raped in prison, or even more, will become pregnant by the enemy, is a very strong theme in the public discourse. I hear it again and again when I lecture about these issues, and in my interviews with soldiers" (personal communication, 1998). The intensity with which the fear of rape of women soldiers is discussed contrasts with the almost total absence of public discussion regarding rape of men in prison, a common and well-documented phenomenon.

Anne Bloom writes, "The prevailing explanation for the IDF's decision to keep women out of actual combat is fear of their being taken prisoner and of possible mistreatment and torture in the hands of the enemy. Yet documentation regarding such incidents is difficult to find" (1993, 137). That the danger of enemy rape is the reason for keeping women out of combat positions is not mentioned in official government documents and is typically hinted at rather than stated outright in public debate (the "various reasons" that we saw earlier). For example, OC Women's Corps Brigadier General Israela Oren urged the IDF to make more jobs available to women and applauded the fact that several combat-related positions had recently opened to women. "Equality is a central value in Israeli society and as one of the main institutions in society we can't ignore this. Still equality cannot come *at any price.* At the moment, I don't see women serving as fighters in the Golani [combat unit]" (*Jerusalem Post,* August 15, 1996; my emphasis).

The press often turns to Yael Rom, the only woman to have flown combat missions in the Sinai campaign in 1956, when the question of women in combat units is raised. Because of her unique role as an Israeli woman combat pilot, Rom's words are imbued with cultural weight. Rom seems to be ever eager to share her views with the Israeli public: She opposes women going into combat not because they cannot handle it, but because of the pressure it would be put on the government to meet ransom demands if a woman combatant were captured. In a recent typical utterance, she pronounced: "'We have to prove that women can do it [fly combat missions], but you have to weigh the cost' she says in a veiled reference to the high ransom price for women taken captive and other dangers for women in combat" (*Jerusalem Post* June 26, 1998).

A similar sentiment was voiced by Prime Minister Rabin when, according to officials in his office, he sought to bury a bill that would enable women to volunteer for combat roles. Rabin opposed the bill at a 1995 cabinet meeting reportedly declaring, "I am totally against this. What happens if a woman falls into captivity? Who will be responsible for *what happens to her?*" (*Jerusalem Post*, February 6, 1995; my emphasis). While not wishing to belittle Rabin's legitimate concern for women in a world filled with gendered violence, one wonders at his choice of words, which seem to suggest that women soldiers, more than men soldiers, are the responsibility of the state. Yet he did not explain why or in what way the state's responsibility for women is greater than for men. Is the IDF not responsible for the safety of its male soldiers, or are men somehow responsible for themselves? Are atrocities committed upon men less atrocious than those committed upon women?

During debates in the Nongovernmental Organizations Forum of the United Nations Conference on Human Rights in Vienna in 1994, human rights activist Rhonda Kopelon addressed these questions from an international perspective, pointing out that rape has been defined by the Geneva Convention as a "crime against honor" rather than as a mode of torture (Yuval-Davis 1997, 110). Kopelon's analysis suggests that what lies behind the determination to keep women out of combat positions is a sense that because women symbolize the collective, rape of a woman—unlike rape or torture of a man—is an affront to the honor of the state. Thus in the Israeli case, if the IDF were to place a woman in a position in which she might be captured and raped by the enemy, the responsibility vis-à-vis the entire Israeli and even the entire Jewish people would be very grave indeed. The rape of a woman soldier is construed as equivalent to the rape of the Jewish people.

The use of the word *rape* to describe what countries at war do to each other reinforces the idea that women's bodies are symbols of the state. Many newspaper articles at the time of the Gulf War talked about the "rape of Kuwait." Sadam Hussein was repeatedly described as an aggressor who ordered "the rape of a tiny, defenseless country." This sort of rhetoric reinforces the notion that men go to war to defend women, and the notion that nations rather than women are the ultimate victims of rape—a misogynistic deceit lethal for women. Those two notions in combination are what drives the wholesale rape of women during wartime. As atrocities in the former Yugoslavia and other situations have shown, armies use rape of women to express conquest of the enemy state (see Brownmiller 1975). By raping what men ostensibly build armies to protect ("womenandchildren"), absolute victory is proclaimed. But more than that, by potentially impregnating the enemies' women, one patriarchal collective truly vanquishes another.

The theme of the capture and rape of women echoes the Biblical story introduced in the epigraph at the start of this section: Dina went out into the land, not only bringing rape upon herself and endangering her menfolk, but also forcing her menfolk to avenge their honor, for which they stooped to the "unmanly" behavior of "unmanning" (that is, circumcising) the enemy—before killing them. More generally, in Jewish culture women's bodies tend to be construed as potentially endangering men. Images of Eve seducing Adam with her fruit and of Delila seducing Samson (and taking away his masculine strength) persist in the cultural imagination in collective concerns with "immodestly" dressed women (see chapter 5) and in fears that the presence of women in combat units would endanger both male soldiers and the purity of the collective. There seems to be no official documentation of the threat of rape to women combatants, perhaps because the IDF is reluctant to open the metamythic discourse of women's bodies as vulnerable and dangerous to intellectual and legal challenge.

Serving in combat has been viewed as the single most important characteristic of a good or perfect Israeli citizen, and women's exclusion from combat has had grave consequences for women's status (see Izraeli 1997). The question of women and combat is complex, predicated on a number of compelling and interlocking cultural understandings that need to be untangled in order to understand what is truly at stake. We have said that Israeli culture presupposes immutable physical differences between men and women. In the best of all cases women fill their "natural" role as mothers, a status that entitles them to protection (and even to collective honor, in the case of grieving mothers of soldiers). Women conscripts in the IDF cannot be mothers (women are dismissed from compulsory service if they become pregnant); motherhood and soldiering are understood to be mutually exclusive national missions. Women soldiers, neither mothers nor true warriors, are in a problematic liminal state. It seems to me that the intense concern with the neatness and sexuality of women soldiers is an expression of that liminality. The "proper" sexuality of the neat and attractive "CHEN" soldier signifies that she is on the appropriate path to suitable motherhood within the collective. The obsessive fear that women soldiers will be raped by the enemy is an expression of the deepest possible threat to patriarchy: that women's motherhood will slip out of the control of the men to whom it "rightfully" belongs.

This fear is continuously restimulated by portrayals of women soldiers that emphasize their sexual attractiveness and sexual vulnerability. These two characteristics become conflated in debates regarding women serving in combat units in the IDF. The public construction of women soldiers as sexy and as beautiful bolsters collective fears that if women were sent into combat they would surely be captured and raped. Juxtaposing rape with feminine beauty and sexuality contributes to the patriarchal deception that women in some way encourage rape, a deception that camouflages the violence underlying patriarchal control of women's bodies.

Rape

Girls Girls

There is no reason to worry [about your impending draft], because the practice in self-defence will help, it turns out, in dates with your boyfriend. —*Quarter Before Joining the Army*

Every man I meet wants to protect me. Can't figure out what from. —MAE WEST

According to police estimates one woman is raped or sexually assaulted every five hours in Israel.
—*Jerusalem Post*, January 27, 1993

Rape is an act of violence and conquest in which gender hierarchy is corporeally constructed and reasserted. And I would argue that rape is an especially effective means of asserting essential corporeal difference. The threat of rape produces gender relations in which women are taught to be dependent upon men to protect them from other men (Griffin 1979). Indeed, the first epigraph in this section relays the dual message that all women are vulnerable to rape, and that all men—even the nice ones ("your boyfriend")—are potential rapists.

A significant body of literature has traced the negative impact of violence and victimization on women's health. I see the link between violence and illness as especially important in the Israeli context, where the culture of gendered militarization means that even those women who are not directly victimized are likely to experience some of the same negative health consequences in their role as grieving mothers of fallen soldiers (see Dyregrov and Matthiesen 1987 on mothers and child-loss) and most especially in their role as potential victims.

Rape survivors exhibit a wide range of emotional and physical symptoms, including sleep and eating disorders, depression, feelings of humiliation, anger, guilt, fear of sex, inability to concentrate, pregnancy, sexually transmitted diseases, suicide, drug and alcohol abuse, hypertension, chronic pelvic pain, irritable bowel syndrome, asthma, and gynecological problems. The World Bank has accumulated substantial proof that the health burden from gender-based victimization among women of reproductive age is equivalent to that of other conditions widely recognized as dangerous for women, such as tuberculosis, cancers, and sepsis during or resulting from birth (Heise 1994, 235). Rape and gendered violence accelerate and intensify the reciprocal construction of femaleness and illness as inherently or "naturally" coinciding conditions.

In Israel, the rhetoric and reality of rape and women's "inherent" weakness, and the rhetoric and reality of women in combat, are mutually constructed in a number of ways. I shall discuss first the public construction of women soldiers as helpless victims with vulnerable bodies. This construction is part of a cultural climate in the IDF that legitimates sexual harassment of women soldiers. I turn from there to reports of regular occurrences of gang rapes in civilian society. Although these are outside the institutional framework of the IDF, the structure of gang rapes parallels the wartime rape of "enemy" women. This message is made explicit in cases in which men's military accomplishments are cited in public and legal discourse as an "excuse" for, or mitigating factor in, rape. The interpenetration of military and civilian violence is even clearer in cases in which weapons distributed by the IDF are used by men to carry out acts of violence, including sexual violence, against women. Finally, I suggest that the public construction of "Woman" as a symbol of the state leads to situations in which actual rapes of real women may be construed as more or less "significant" depending upon the extent to which particular women are assimilated to the national symbolic "Woman."

The Public Construction of Women Soldiers as Helpless Victims with Vulnerable Bodies

While Israel lays claim to being the only nation in the contemporary world that has institutionalized conscription of women into military service, the military training women receive does not (usually) empower them to defend themselves, much less to defend their country. Quite to the contrary, the IDF often seems to train women to be, or at least to see themselves as, victims rather than aggressors. During basic training, young women receive minimal instruction in firing weapons, just enough to give them a "feel" for what the army is; it does not enable them to use the weapons to defend themselves or their country. Women recruits are told about the dangers of rape—to be careful at night and to report sexual harassment—yet they are not given the tools to protect themselves from rape or other forms of violence. Most women soldiers receive only five lessons in self-defense during their three-week basic training. Discussions of the danger of rape without the training or weapons to fight rape can be seen as grooming women for corporeal fear.

The image of women soldiers as victims is rarely contradicted in public presentations. Women soldiers are almost never shown in poses suggesting strength or assertiveness, but rather, as Edna Levy-Schreiber has documented, in poses of neatness and prettiness. The vulnerability of women soldiers has been on the public agenda many times over the years. Following several "incidents" in 1983, newspapers reported that the IDF decided to arm women soldiers with tear gas. While the uninitiated might infer that the IDF wanted to train women soldiers to fight the enemy, Israeli readers would have understood that the presumed attackers were actually Israeli men and that the goal of the IDF program was to allow women to escape rather than to fight back. Apparently oblivious to the irony of the situation they created, the IDF explained that the trial program of giving tear gas to 10% of women soldiers was necessary because the army relies on hitchhiking to get troops around the country, but most female soldiers hold administrative posts so they do not travel armed and therefore are particularly exposed to assault (*Jerusalem Post*, September 25, 1983).

Ten years later the IDF considered giving women soldiers new self-defense devices. Although they already had small tear gas canisters, it turned out that the women almost never used them. The new plan was to give them electric shockers or colored spray that remains on an attacker's face for eight hours, both of which, it was presumed, women soldiers would be less afraid to use than tear gas. In addition, the IDF forbid women soldiers to hitchhike after dark and instructed them to hitchhike during the day only together with a male soldier (*Jerusalem Post*, March 17, 1993), policies that did little to empower women.

Those (few) women soldiers who do receive useful military training understand the connection between rape and the insufficient training most other women receive. And they understand that Israeli women are most likely to be attacked by Israeli men, not by the amorphous "enemy." Hanna Shimon, who was interviewed after graduating at the top of her platoon, told a reporter that "If I were attacked by a rapist in a dark alley, I would know how to deal with him. Instinctively, I would choke him, one blow and he'd get the message. He'd find out he's not dealing with a loser" (*Jerusalem Post*, June 7, 1996). Her declaration implies that the majority of women soldiers, who do not receive the extra training that Shimon received, are just that—losers.

When incidents of rape are reported in Israeli newspapers, the profession or occupation of the victim is rarely mentioned (the detail most often mentioned seems to be the victim's age). An exception to the norm is cases in which the victim is a woman soldier, whether or not the rape occurred within the framework of her IDF service. This practice contributes to the construction of women soldiers as "rape-able"—that is, as attractive and vulnerable victims of male sexual aggression. In one article we learn that a fifteen-year-old boy climbed over the gate of a base where a woman soldier was on guard duty, grabbed her by the throat, stole her Uzi submachine gun, ripped off her shirt looking for ammunition, cut her with a pocket knife, and attempted to rape her. He fled with the Uzi after tying her up with her shoelaces (*Jerusalem Post*, April 8, 1991). The images that this report conjures are not likely to contribute to the sense of empowerment of women soldiers. But even more shocking, there were no editorials in the paper that week questioning why the training received by women soldiers is so poor that even with a submachine gun this soldier could not defend herself against a fifteen-year-old boy with a pocket knife.[14]

In an examination of the history of women and combat in the British armed forces, Cynthia Enloe makes the important point that women have not always been kept away from locations of danger; navy commanders sent women nurses to the South Atlantic as part of the Falklands task force, knowing that their ships could be attacked as easily as any other ships (1983, 154–155). Women have served as spies, even crossing into enemy territory, a situation of extreme personal danger (Quester 1982, 226). And in modern wars, civilians tend to be in as much danger as soldiers, civilian status did not protect Vietnamese women from rape by American soldiers or Croatian women from rape by Serbian soldiers. Mady Segal notes that in the American military women are placed in combat zones but in defensive capacities only.

> Women in specialities such as tank turret repairman, radar technician, long-range missile crewman, and military police (to name a few) can be expected to be in battle. Even women in the "traditional" female specialities, such as the medical and administrative ones, may still be in the line of fire. Thus, we allow women to be in positions where they can be killed by enemy fire, but we bar them from those positions in which they can initiate attack. (Segal 1982, 268)

Where many armies seem to draw the line, Enloe, Segal, and Jeff Tuten all explain, is at giving women weapons. The examples they cite suggest that while distancing women from danger is indeed a fundamental reason for excluding women from combat positions, distancing women from possessing weapons may be even more fundamental.[15]

A Cultural Climate in the IDF That Legitimates Sexual Harassment of Women Soldiers

My Sister the Soldier

Yes, I have a sister, a soldier sister. A "babe" who confuses everyone. On the street people always look at her. Her uniform, it turns out, is flattering to her. And if high-ranking officers come to our house, clearly that is because of my sister's braids, and don't tell me that it is because of her special job that they always need her, "stat" and right away. Yes I have a soldier sister and through her I get to know the army in an unconventional way. Once an officer from the Air Force came by who had to pass some secret message through her. And once a Navy officer came to ask if the old message is still around. And once for a reconnaissance drill a Maintenance Corps officer dropped by. And then she had a tip dropped by a young officer from the Communication Corps. And it is clear to me that it is for her and not for me that almost the whole General Staff visited our house. And not one officer from this select group could understand that my sister has a boyfriend in the Commandos, a corporal or a sergeant, stern-faced. I tell you, he is quite a guy. One day he told me, when you get your draft notice, don't hesitate to call me, and I will explain the army to you, and all of that because you have a great sister . . ."

—*Quarter Before Joining the Army,* facing a picture of a woman soldier in uniform sitting in front of a mirror, with cosmetics on a table, putting on lipstick

Sexual harassment of women soldiers takes a variety of forms in the IDF, and is so widespread as to be all but unremarkable. It is common for male soldiers to shout sexual invitations and comments at women soldiers, and while the extent of this behavior varies from unit to unit it is an acknowledged part of IDF culture. Moreover, it seems to be the case that sexual harassment is seen as a problem that women in the IDF need to learn to cope with, rather than as a practice that men need to learn to refrain from. According to *HaAretz* (October 14, 1999), the IDF refused to authorize a class on preventing violence against women for male recruits even though it has agreed to run the program for female recruits. In interviews conducted with women soldiers by Orna Sasson-Levy, incidents were repeatedly mentioned that sounded to Sasson-Levy like sexual harassment, yet were dismissed as *k'taim* [practical jokes] or "trivial" by women soldiers. One informant told Sasson-Levy that when the male soldiers she worked with were annoyed at her they would sing: "Ruti is a whore, Ruti sucks off the whole platoon." Significantly, Sasson-Levy's informants, exceptional young women serving in traditional male roles in the IDF, disclosed that they would not report sexual harassment because they would not want to be perceived as victims. One said she would not want to be seen acting "like a girl." Ambiguous in her comments is whether "acting like a girl" means being a victim of sexual harassment, or turning to authority figures for protection from sexual harassment. It likely means both.

Simona Sharoni observes that the militarization of Israeli society was ushered in and embodied by the charismatic Moshe Dayan, who in 1953 was named commander in chief of the IDF. He became a symbol of the *sabra*:

militant, arrogant, and exceedingly masculine . . . Dayan emerged as a primary role model for Jewish men, representing a shift from a past of perceived helplessness

> and powerlessness associated with the European-Jewish experience to a present and future of personal and military prowess and strength. Jewish manhood had been redeemed and redefined in terms of an aggressively militarized national state. (1995, 96)[16]

In the popular imagination, Dayan is not only the symbol of the *sabra* par excellence but also the prototypical soldier-lover, renowned for his sexual liaisons at a time in which sexual relations between male officers and their female clerks were commonplace (*HaAretz*, March 19, 1999). The admixture of traits that Dayan symbolizes constructs an Israeli male who is strong, healthy, brave, experienced at combat, and sexually predatory. In light of cultural understandings of gender as a dichotomous system, we may ask where this amalgam leaves women.

In a study carried out in the United States by Peggy Crull (1984), 45% of women who had been sexually harassed at work reported that the harassment interfered with their ability to carry out their jobs. Many women began to doubt their own abilities and question their career choices; 94% of sexually harassed women in her sample reported stress symptoms. Many also reported anger, fear, depression, embarrassment, sleeplessness, and guilt. Approximately 36% of the women pointed out physical ailments that they thought had been brought on by sexual harassment. Most common were nausea, fatigue, headaches, weight change, and generally lowered resistance to illness. Sexual harassment, in other words, perpetuates a cycle in which women, already perceived as vulnerable (otherwise their harassers would be more wary), are weakened and sickened, made even more vulnerable, and thus "legitimately" excluded from positions of leadership and authority.

The newspaper *Ma'ariv* reported in 1993 that there are approximately one thousand cases of sexual harassment in the IDF each year but only about 10% reach the level where they are investigated. (The IDF has not been particularly forthcoming with statistics on sexual harassment; see Barnoy 1997, 86). As the general social climate in Israel has begun to encourage women to report abuse, the number of sexual harassment complaints investigated by the military police has risen, up 43% in 1998 from the 1997 figure. OC Women's Corps Brigadier General Orit Adato reported to the Knesset Committee on the Status of Women that this means that complaints are taken more seriously: Twenty-three indictments were served in 1998, only sixteen in 1997. (I do not see this as a significant change.) Adato noted that one in three complaints was of a physical attack, the rest of verbal harassment. Most cases resulting in indictments, however, were of physical attacks, a record that perpetuates the culture of shouting sexual invitations and insults at women soldiers (*Jerusalem Post*,

January 20, 1999). Verbal abuse is a particularly insidious form of gendered violence; it is often dismissed as "trivial" and its perpetrators go unpunished, leaving the victim without even the consolation of having her feelings of fear and humiliation legitimated by society. Verbal abuse also serves as a reminder of the threat of rape: Women experience sexual harassment as frightening precisely because the words carry with them a reminder that all women in patriarchal societies are "rape-able."

According to Brigadier General Adato, the IDF's policy is that a soldier may not ask to be transferred to another unit on the basis of a sexual harassment incident unless she agrees to file a complaint. While this policy ostensibly encourages women to pursue charges against offending men, I suspect that in the highly gendered power structure of the IDF it can be difficult for women to file complaints against their superior officers. Thus this policy may actually force women victims of sexual harassment into staying on the base in which the harassment occurred or continues to occur. The issue of hierarchy is indeed relevant: Adato reported the breakdown by rank of those accused of sexual harassment: 27% conscripts, 24% career soldiers, *28% officers*, 7% civilian workers, 4% reservists, 10% not specified (*Jerusalem Post*, January 20, 1999; my emphasis).[17]

Peggy Crull has argued that, "Sexual harassment grows out of the economic and psychological inequality between the sexes that is built into the workforce as well as the whole culture and is reinforced by the class system that pervades every institution of our society" (1984, 102). Men hold higher status jobs, have more formal training, more seniority, are more likely to be in unions and to be closely connected with old boys' networks that protect them from complaints of sexual harassment (this last is doubly true of the IDF). "Indeed, sexual harassment may be a demonstration of that status and power, and not primarily motivated by sexual feelings. It may also be a route through which men bolster class and status differences among themselves" (102), a pattern that could explain the high rate of male officers among those who sexually harass women soldiers.

The IDF's response to sexual harassment has changed over the years. Until the mid-1990s, the prevalent attitude seems to have been one of nonchalance, particularly when the culprit was an officer and the victim was a conscript serving under him. In the mid-1980s when two women soldiers complained of sexual harassment, IDF spokesman Brigadier General Ephraim Lapid responded:

> We get involved only when there is a crime or prominent wrongdoing. We cannot respond regarding voluntary sexual relations, as in the IDF there also are young single officers who develop positive relationships with the women soldiers with whom they work. Also when the man is married and the woman soldier gives in to

> his wooing, we have no control over that. We must remember that there have also been cases of unjustified complaints made by women soldiers, and these caused injustice to the officers. The social fortitude of the army is a value in Israel's security. We should not ignore injury to the individual in the military community, but it is also wrong to blow this topic out of proportion. (*HaAretz*, March 20, 1985; cited in Barnoy 1997, 84)

A case that in the eyes of many in the IDF community was "blown out of proportion" concerns Brigadier General Nir Galili, who had been found having sexual intercourse with the woman soldier who served as his personal assistant in 1995–1996 at an army base in Tze'elim. At the time, she lodged a complaint that he had sexual relations with her and raped her, and Galili was tried by a disciplinary court and found guilty of conduct unbecoming an officer.[18] It was ruled that he could not be promoted for two years, a period that ended in April 1998. In early 1999 the IDF announced his promotion to major-general and appointment as commander of a key field division. The woman (now former) soldier petitioned the High Court, asking for an injunction stopping the promotion. She claimed that from the beginning Galili ought to have been court-martialed rather than chastised for "inappropriate sexual behavior" by a disciplinary court. She charged that the IDF had put improper pressure on her in order to avoid court-martialing Galili. At the time of the incident she was nineteen years old and sexually inexperienced, and he was forty, married, and a father of three. According to the former soldier, chief IDF prosecutor General Uri Shoham had decided not to remove Galili from the IDF even though he knew she was not Galili's only victim (*HaAretz*, March 10, 1999).

The defense offered by Galili's friends and lawyer centered upon his military accomplishments, a discursive technique that constructed the State and women's bodies as opposing values. Galili's lawyer declared, "Galili is a senior officer, learned in battle and difficult conditions. Yet the battle for his good name and proving his ability to continue to contribute to the security of the country is his most difficult yet" (*HaAretz*, March 10, 1999). The lawyer argued that Galili had already been promoted twice since the original punishment, and that two defense ministers (Moshe Arens and Yitzhak Mordechai, who, in April 2000, the police recommended charging on multiple counts of sexual abuse of women working under him) and two Chiefs of Joint Staff (Amnon Shahak and Shaul Mofaz) had decided to promote him despite what had happened with the woman soldier (*HaAretz*, March 26, 1999). In sum since the highest authorities in the IDF thought that sexually abusing a young woman soldier should not prevent promotion, it would be inappropriate for the court to rule otherwise.

Throughout the case, Chief of Joint Staff Major General Shaul Mofaz reiterated that Galili is an excellent officer whose appointment is very important to the security of the country. Mofaz wrote in his deposition to the court: "I took exception to and I condemned Galili's behavior. But as the Commander of the IDF I cannot turn my attention away from the fundamental matter: The supreme need that on the day of reckoning [*yom p'kuda*] the safety of the soldiers and the citizens will be in the hands of the best officers" (*HaAretz*, March 29, 1999). Implying that delays in appointing Galili threaten national security (or, put differently, that prosecuting a man for raping a young woman under his command threatens national security), Mofaz explained that Galili is the best candidate for the position. "Changing the situation at the last minute [before a planned large-scale maneuver drill] will undermine the expected appointment and will force the system to change the appointment protocol, and that will hurt the functioning of the army and its expected operational activities" (*HaAretz*, March 12, 1999).

In a decision that surprised many Israelis and dismayed part of the IDF community, the High Court ruled in late March 1999 that Galili cannot be promoted. He was not, however, removed from command or asked to leave the IDF.

Military Accomplishments, Collective Violence, and Rape

1990: Several gang rapes involving school-age rapists and victims reported in Petach Tikvah.
1993: Town in the North. Twenty youths raped a fourteen-year-old girl.
1993: Haifa area. Seven youths repeatedly gang raped a fourteen-year-old girl from their school.
1993: Six men raped a volunteer on a moshav in the Arava.
1994: Eleven boys at Kibbutz Shomrat raped a fourteen-year-old girl.
1995: Five young men from the town of Sderot raped, sodomized, and abused a mentally handicapped sixteen-year-old girl.
1995: Three Kiryat Ata men who gang-raped a mentally retarded women over a period of several months were sentenced in Haifa to three to six months of community service and two years' suspended sentence.
1995: Five youths from Kiryat Gat gang-raped a fifteen-year-old girl at knifepoint.
1997: Beer Sheva region. Four youths gang-raped a fifteen-year-old girl. The Beer Sheva District Court ordered a lighter sentence for one of the rapists because, according to the court, he was the last to rape her and by that point did not have to use force.
1998: Seven youths from Daliat al-Carmel and Usfiya charged with rape and aggravated assault.

(All reports gleaned from Israeli newspapers.)

Accounts of gang rapes appear regularly in the Israeli press. Because most rapes go unreported,[19] and because the press elects to run articles about only those rapes it considers "newsworthy," I cannot know whether gang rapes are more common in Israel than in other societies. (The one statistic I could get hold of is from the Association of Rape Crisis Centers in Israel, which reports that in 1998 out of 5,236 calls regarding sexual attacks, 170 reported gang rapes). But I do know it is important to think about gang rapes in the context of the militarization of gendered bodies. First, gang rapes parallel military operations in the male communal structure of the acts of violence. Second, as we shall see, certain gang rapes in Israel are "forgiven" because of military associations.

Late in 1998 a high school girl was repeatedly gang raped by a group of fellow students, young men between the ages of fifteen and seventeen in the town of Ramat HaSharon—a town considered to be something of a model Israeli community. Unless otherwise noted, my analysis here relies upon the in-depth report published by Esti Aharonovitch in *Ma'ariv*, *Sof Shavua'* (January 1, 1999).

During the course of visits and interviews in the town and school, Aharonovitch witnessed a public reaction highly colored by military culture. Gabi Paran, the recently elected head of the local council (equivalent to a municipal or a district council in other countries), called the rapes "an operational accident in an elite [fighting] unit." To Aharonovitch, these words made it seem "as if the rape suspects and the youth and their compatriots were a Commando unit on its way to an operation in Lebanon when they were ambushed by the Hizbullah." The high school principal asked reporters why they don't write about the good things in his school, "like the art club." As Aharonovitch was leaving the school, she saw the principal running to catch up with her. "You see that group of boys over there. They are preparing to be in shape for combat units, we have a club for that. At our school, everyone goes to combat units." The principal, vice-principal, and other officials of the town boastfully reiterated that their town produces more pilots for the IDF than any other town in Israel.[20] Months later the father of one of the ringleaders was quoted saying about his son, "This is a boy you can trust from A to Z, a boy whose dream was to study law and go into an elite commando unit" (*HaAretz*, September 3, 1999).

The sentiments expressed by the principal and head of the local council were shared by much of the community. While a few of the victim's female friends have stood by her, much of the school and town seems to be standing behind the rapists. High school students even tried to organize a bus to go and support the boys who had been arrested. Students with information about the rapes were afraid to come forward—they were intimidated by the rapists' friends—and the young woman who was raped has been threatened with violence if she returns to school. In a reversal that may be difficult for outsiders to comprehend, the boys have come to be seen as victims and the victim has come to be seen as the culprit.

If boys who rape should be forgiven because they serve (or will serve, or might serve) in elite military units, girls can be blamed for provoking male sexual attention. The boys are victims, the community claims, of the "sluttish" behavior of the raped girl. Aharonovitch talked to youths in the school. "One boy said: She is a liar. You should see how she puts on cosmetics. Another said: I am angry at her. I am really pissed off. How she got us in trouble like this. She wanted it." In a comment that reveals the interpenetration of traditional and modern-consumer patriarchal narratives, one of her female classmates blamed her, saying, "Everyday her hair was a different color, perms, short skirts, rib shirts . . ." (*HaAretz*, September 3, 1999). The mother of two of the rapists said, "If I had known what was going on [in her son's bedroom the night several boys raped and threatened the victim with a knife] I would have kicked her out of the house . . . this will cost her dearly. How [did she have the nerve] to seduce my sons." The father of one of the boys defended his son saying he is a "good kid" and didn't know that what he did was against the law. "If they bring you a woman and say 'take her,' what, you won't take her?" When pressed by the reporter the father answered that, "Everything is in God's hands. It was a moment's temptation." And the father of another one of the boys boasted, "I spent fifteen years in prison and I've showered in a lot of places, but I've never seen a 'tool' as big as the one my son has on him anywhere. If he had forced her, nothing would have been left of her" (*HaAretz*, September 3, 1999).

The victim understood that she would be blamed for the rapes, and that is the reason she did not tell anyone of her ordeal until she reached a state of collapse. In her report to the police she explained that the threat the boys held over her was that if she did not cooperate with them or if she told anyone what they were doing, they would spread it around that school that she was a "slut." The use of gendered terrorism of this sort worked so well because the patriarchal system constructs women as vulnerable, and then offers to defend only those women who meet certain (sometimes ephemeral) standards. Perhaps most shocking, according to Aharonovitch, is that the repeated gang rapes of a high school student elicited little public dismay and soon disappeared from the newspapers. No one seemed to wonder whether there might, after all, be some connection between a community culture that raises boys for the commandos, and a community culture that turns a blind eye to sexual violence. While the case of Ramat HaSharon is unusually horrific, it is an exaggeration of social patterns found elsewhere in Israel rather than an exception to those patterns. The idealization of militarism dictates a teen culture inclined to violence. And indeed, of twenty-three European countries participating in a study of youth behavior, Israel ranked number one in rates of teen violence among boys (not among girls; Harel 1999).

In August 1999 the rapists—whose names were never revealed to the press—were convicted as juveniles. On December 15, 1999, the seven teenage boys were sentenced, three to prison terms ranging from two and one-half to four years and the remaining four to community service. As he gave the sentences, Judge Natan Amit explained that "The defendents have learned nothing. They continue to stand by their claim that they are the real victims of the whole affair . . . and their families also support this position." An evaluation of the victim submitted to the court describes her, since the rape, as rarely leaving her house, unable to trust anybody, and suffering from acute insomnia and nightmares (*HaAretz*, December 16, 1999).

Use of Weapons Distributed by the IDF to Carry Out Acts of Violence against Women

According to some estimates, one out of every seven women in Israel is subjected to some sort of physical violence at some point in her life (Yishai 1997, 198). Violence against women is not unique to Israel, and Israel rightfully boasts rape crisis hotlines, community police officers trained to work with rape victims, shelters for battered women, even a hostel for men who batter, and laws that prohibit sexual and domestic violence. But Israel does have the special problem of IDF weapons.

In late December 1998 three Israeli women were murdered and one wounded by men who held legal gun permits. In the most publicized of the cases, Shoshana Tsabari was murdered by her husband six months after she had asked for a restraining order to distance her husband from the house, and the judge had refused the request saying that in her opinion Shoshana was lying. What I wish to draw attention to is that the M-16 assault rifle with which Shlomo Tsabari murdered his wife and then committed suicide was handed to him by his reserve unit in the IDF. Apparently, while it sometimes happens that the IDF is notified of criminal proceedings against a soldier and his reserve duty is deferred so as not to give him a weapon, other times the IDF is not informed. According to reports in the press, there is no orderly system at work that prevents men known to be violent from returning home with IDF weapons (*Jerusalem Post*, January 2, 1998).

Deputy Commander Ido Gutman, head of the police patrol division that deals with approving gun permits for the Ministry of the Interior, explained that there is an arrangement by which the police notify the IDF regarding dangerous citizens only when they are convicted or when there are "a large number of complaints" against them. The IDF is an autonomous body not subordinate to either the police or the Ministry of the Interior; in principle, the IDF can decide to give weapons to a man accused of domestic or other forms of violence,

> if the IDF feels [the man] must have a weapon to perform his assigned task . . . Everyone is very sensitive about this issue. It isn't just the women's groups who are concerned. But there are limitations regarding restrictions. Let's assume that some twenty women are killed each year by people who hold gun permits. What are we going to do? Stop giving permits? Then we'd have an absurd situation where you'd have unarmed guards at schools and a terrorist could come in and kill a whole classroom. Then what would Ms. [Ofra] Friedman [chairwoman of Na'amat, the women's branch of the Histadrut Labor Organization] say? (*Jerusalem Post*, January 1, 1998).

In his statement, Deputy Commander Gutman constructed a very particular sort of gendered corporeal schema. Not only did he subsume women's safety to national security, but he justified writing off the lives of women ("some twenty women are killed each year") by weighing women against children ("terrorists could come in and kill a whole classroom.") While I would never suggest that the remarks of one individual represent the sentiments of an entire country, it must be remembered that Gutman is a high-ranking officer in the police department. His remarks reveal what is usually obscured and concealed in the rhetoric of war "on behalf of womenandchildren": "Womenandchildren" is a trope for the (male-dominated) collective, and when push comes to shove, women may be disposable.

The climate of war is not conducive to women's health or safety. During the Gulf War there was a steady increase in the number of incidents of murder and battering of women by their spouses (Deutsch 1994, 102). This increase is typically attributed to the stress felt by brave Israeli men forced to "impotently" sit out the Gulf War (Israel agreed to refrain from active involvement in order to allow the United States to build a coalition that included Arab countries). I believe this view to be myopic in the extreme. Cultures of violence feed on acts of violence. For women, the side on which the armed man is ostensibly fighting may make little difference. Simona Sharoni (1994) cites the appalling case of Gilad Shemen, who, during military service in the Gaza Strip in 1989, shot and killed a seventeen-year-old Palestinian woman who was sitting and reading a book on her front porch. Two years later he shot and killed his former girlfriend, nineteen-year-old Einav Rogel, who had stuck by him during his trial over the Gaza shooting, even though he had been violently abusing her at the time.

The IDF is not the only Israeli institution that facilitates violence against women. It should be seen as a central but not exclusive player in constructing and preserving a culture in which violence against women is insufficiently discouraged, and sometimes actually encouraged, by public institutions. State-supported, all-male, Orthodox rabbinical courts—holding a monopoly on divorce under Israeli law—often seem to be more concerned with keeping the family together (what they call "*sh'lom bayit,*" conjugal harmony) than with protecting women from violent husbands. Studies show that half of battered women who had taken refuge in shelters and sued their husbands in rabbinic court were told to return home for *sh'lom bayit* (Swirski 1991, 324). The civil courts do not seem to be of much more help to women. On August 3, 1999, three domestic violence cases were reported in the *Jerusalem Post*. In one case a man threatened to murder his wife, and choked, slapped, and scratched her. The woman told the court that this was not the first time he had attacked her. The judge released him on 1,500 shekels (approximately 400 dollars) bail and barred him from going near his wife for fifteen days. A second man who beat his wife and threatened her in front of the police was also released on 1,500 shekels bail. A third man who threatened to stab his sister-in-law to death was also released on 1,500 shekels bail. The bargain price of 1,500 shekels for a woman seems to belie claims by IDF officers and government officials that the "price" of women serving in combat (that is, the risk of capture and rape) is too high.

Public Constructions of Women as Symbols of the State

> Our little land
> Our pretty land
> Motherland [*moledet*] without a night shirt
> Barefoot motherland
> Accept me unto your songs
> Beautiful bride
> Open your gates
> I will come, I will praise God
>
> Song by Yoram Tahalov,
> performed by pop star Rami Kleinstein

The rape of certain women in Israel is regarded as more "significant" than the rape of other women. In 1998 Linor Abergil, the reigning "Miss Israel" who was later crowned "Miss World," was raped while in Italy. Her symbolic status as Miss Israel seems to have led the press and the public to interpret the rape in collective rather than merely personal terms: Whoever raped her, raped Israel. The rapist was at first described in the Israeli press as an Egyptian; then he was described as an Egyptian who had moved to Israel; in fact, as later press reports revealed, his name is Uri Shlomo and he is a Jewish Israeli travel agent who, parenthetically, was born in Egypt. Still, he is consistently referred to in the press as an "Egyptian-born Israeli," although it is most unusual for Israeli Jews to be described in the Israeli press in terms of their place of birth (unless it is somehow relevant to the matter at hand). What I am suggesting is that when a national symbol is raped, the rape is easily interpreted in nationalist terms. Linor Abergil was turned into one more victim in the Israeli-Arab war, a sleight of hand that disguised the gendered violence that underpins beauty contests, reinforced popular beliefs that beautiful women incite uncontrollable lust in men, and fed into public fears of the enemy raping "our" women. If the rapist could be identified as an Arab, then Miss Israel's body is truly the national body. On December 29, 1999, the man who raped Linor Abergil was sentenced to sixteen years imprisonment, twelve years more than the maximum sentence received by the ringleader of the Ramat HaSharon gang of rapists.

In case the significance of the rape of a national symbol eluded public understanding, the point was clarified when the next Miss Israel was selected. In March 1999 the television and newspapers were filled with exciting news: For the first time in Israeli history an Israeli Arab, Rena Resslan, had been chosen to be Miss Israel and represent Israel in the Miss World competition. Given the timing, one cannot but wonder whether the national crown was worth just a bit less after it had been raped. One more bit of news underscored the institutional competition and collusion in matters of female corporeality: A few months earlier Natrofil Medikacenter, a chain of hair removal clinics, had signed Rena Resslan, at a low rate of pay, for a year of advertising aimed at the Arab sector. The company announced that it had no intention of releasing the new Miss Israel from her contract, although *LaIsha*, the women's magazine that sponsors the competition, does not permit its beauty queens to appear in advertisements for one year after the coronation. As of mid-March 1999, just two weeks after Prime Minister Netanyahu announced that the selection of an Arab for the Miss Israel title proves that there is equality and coexistence between Jews and Arabs in Israel, Natrofil Medikacenter and *LaIsha* were fighting over who would profit first from the new Miss Israel's body (*Kol HaIr*, March 12, 1999). For women in Israel, even winning can feel like losing.

Interestingly, the press published sporadic comments linking the Nir Galili case to the case of Linor Abergil (the two high-profile rape cases of the season), in that both Linor Abergil and the former soldier were brave enough to make their own stories public and thereby encourage other women rape victims to come forth (*HaAretz*, March 23, 1999). But I think the link between the two cases is much greater. Both victims belong to the category of especially "rape-able" women—a beauty queen and a woman soldier. Both cases have to do with the rape of symbols of the collective. And both cases ended on ambiguous notes: Abergil's successor as Miss Israel is an Arab whose body is now being exploited by a hair removal company, and Galili continues to receive some degree of public support and still serves as an officer in the IDF.

Not all rape victims in Israel are treated with as much sympathy as Miss Israel. Another Israeli woman and "Egyptian" man were involved in a situation in which the outcome was far different. In November 1998 Shlomit Shalom, an Israeli belly dancer, protested in front of the Foreign Ministry demanding that the government send home Egyptian ambassador Mohammed Bassiouny, whom she accused of sexually attacking her in August 1997. The criminal case against him had been dismissed by the court. She had then filed for civil damages, but the court ruled that Bassiouny had diplomatic immunity. With a clear understanding of the issues involved, Shalom commented that "Israel should not sacrifice the rights of women for a diplomatic relationship with a foreign country" (*Jerusalem Post*, November 12, 1998). Significantly, at the time of the court case a gag order was placed barring publication of details of the attempted rape. Attorneys of the Foreign Ministry had requested the gag order saying that Israeli embassy personnel in Cairo could be harmed if the incident continued to be reported abroad, and that Israel's relations with Egypt were on the verge of collapse over this case.

Ironically, in a country that has made a systematic project of keeping women out of combat units because of the risk of rape at the hands of the enemy, a woman who actually accused an "enemy" of attempting to rape her was shushed by her own government. In part, this incident suggests once again that in situations in which the interests of women oppose the interests of the state, when push comes to shove it is the woman who is pushed and shoved. Yet I think that in this particular incident an additional factor was at work—the profession of the woman involved. As a belly dancer (and that is how she was designated in virtually all of the newspaper reports, although with the exception of "soldier," the profession of women rape victims is rarely mentioned in the press) she abdicated her "right" to be protected along with "womenandchildren."

Rape of women who symbolize the collective is intolerable, but rape of women who do not is somehow, sometimes, not quite so bad. While official documentation is sketchy, there is much anecdotal information suggesting that when Russian immigrants are raped, public response is colored by the popular belief that "all Russian women are prostitutes." It is certainly the case that trafficking in women from the former Soviet Union has elicited far less public censure than the rape of Linor Abergil. For example, Petia Pinhasov, a "Russian Mafia" leader, was sentenced to just fifteen years in jail for brutally beating and raping women brought over as virtual slaves from the former Soviet Union and forced to work in massage parlors. Other gang members were sentenced to even shorter terms of imprisonment (seven months to four years) on counts of violence and abduction, and two gang members were released when Judge Uri Strusman determined they were not hardened criminals and had already served sufficient time while in custody awaiting trial (*Jerusalem Post*, July 13, 1993).

A Truly Vicious Cycle

In a study of the consequences of a history of victimization among women members of a health maintenance organization, Mary Koss (1994) found that criminal victimization was a more important factor in predicting physician visits than marital status, age, or other known health hazards. The mean number of outpatient visits in the year of the study exactly mirrored the severity of prior victimization: Each increment in severity was associated with an increase of 33% in physician visits.[21] Koss's study quantifies the extent to which harm inflicted upon women in the context of one patriarchal institution tends to force them into dependency upon another patriarchal institution. The social processes of militarization and gendered violence lead not only to illness but also to the medicalization of women's bodies. Koss has described a sickening scenario in which women suffer somatically from the male-dominated culture of violence, and then submit to the authority figures of the male-dominated medical establishment in order to be "cured" of their symptoms.

Violence indeed makes women sick, but medical treatment does little more than disguise the true source of illness by training ever more attention upon women's "pathological" bodies rather than upon the truly pathological cultural patterns that make violence and gender hierarchy seem inevitable. I have argued in this chapter that the militarization of Israeli society constructs an imperfect and vulnerable female body. This conceptualization is a necessary part of the military project: It both justifies the righteousness of war (to protect "womenandchildren") and provides an omnipresent "Other" over and against which the male-warrior can self-define. Women are conscripted into this project through cultural devices that create "rape-able" female bodies. The outcome is a circular schema in which rape, violence, and the threat of rape and violence make women sick and weak; sick and weak women understand themselves to be dependent upon healthy and strong men to defend them; healthy and strong men need to defend women from the everpresent threat of enemy men who would rob women of the sexual purity that symbolizes the national collective; sexual purity is valuable only in a noticeably attractive (thin, neat, delicate, desirable) female body; attractive female bodies are construed as the "cause" of gendered violence; and gendered violence makes women sick.

Chapter 4

The Ritualized Body

Brides, Purity, and the Mikveh

For discourse is not only an instrument of persuasion, operating along rational (or pseudo-rational) and moral (or pseudo-moral) lines, but it is also an instrument of sentiment evocation. Moreover, it is through these paired instrumentalities—ideological persuasion and sentiment evocation—that discourse holds the capacity to shape and reshape society itself.

—Bruce Lincoln, *Discourse and the Construction of Society*

For three sins women die in the hour of giving birth: For carelessness in keeping *niddah* [laws of menstrual purity], *challah* [removing a portion of dough as tithe to the priesthood], and [Shabbat] candle-lighting.

—Mishnah Shabbat 2:6

This chapter focuses on a setting—the mikveh—in which the gendered corporeal themes that we have been looking at throughout this book are ritualized. The mikveh is a purificatory ritual bath primarily used by women in conjunction with menstrual and childbirth bleeding. Popular discourses regarding niddah (menstrual impurity, which is resolved through immersion in the mikveh) and ceremonial prenuptial immersion in the mikveh demonstrate how rituals work on sensory and corporeal levels to create effects that seem "really real" (Geertz 1973). By engaging in the intimate corporeal drills of the niddah-mikveh ritual sequence, Jewish Israeli women reenact or reembody events, values, stories, and symbols of cultural significance, thus drawing themselves into (or being drawn into) collective narratives of gender and purity.

Attention to ritual is of crucial importance because, as Bruce Lincoln has shown so well, hierarchies (including gender hierarchies) are established and defended, "through those discourses that legitimate or mystify their structures, premises, and workings" (1989, 173). Symbolic discourses such as ritual, myth, spectacle, gesture, costume, and icon obviate the need for the direct use of coercive force, which anyway remains "a stopgap measure: effective in the short run, unworkable over the long haul," and transform simple power into legitimate authority (4–5).[1] Hierarchies certainly make use of physical coercion and rational persuasion, but more than that hierarchies are created and sustained by authority—by "a posited, perceived, or institutionally ascribed asymmetry"—that permits certain people to command the confidence, respect, and trust of others, or "an important proviso—to make [others] act *as if* this were so" (Lincoln 1994, 4). Ritual contexts, with their suspension of rational questioning and their aura of divine directive, authenticity, and tradition, are especially potent frameworks for forging relationships of authority and subordination.

In Israeli society, as in much of the world, control of women's bodies is enacted as much through symbolic discourses and ritual performances as through direct expressions of power. The "advantage" of symbolic control is that it has the capacity to evoke feelings of allegiance and loyalty among those who might seem (to outsiders) to have a great deal to lose from cooperating with authoritarian institutions. The "problem" with symbolic control is that it tends not to be absolute or complete; it continuously needs to be reenacted, inspected, scrutinized, checked, and double-checked. This pattern of surveillance, epitomized in the Jewish-Israeli niddah and mikveh ritual complex, has some very serious corporeal consequences for women. By encouraging women and men to pay excessive attention to women's bodies, women come to be seen as "more bodily" than men. This collective perception feeds into a gendered conceptual schema in which men are construed as associated with projects of culture, while women are construed as mired in their own corporeality (Ortner 1996). Because culture is by definition "above" nature (the process of making culture is the process of conquering nature), this conceptualization further legitimates social programs of controlling (socializing or enculturing) women's bodies.

In many cultures, including Israel, men and women believe that women's bodies in their normal state are "too" natural. In the particular Jewish-Israeli version, the hypernaturalness of women's bodies tends to be interpreted as illness, weakness, vulnerability, or niddah, and tends to be "treated" through the expert care of physicians, politicians, and rabbis who sometimes collude and sometimes compete for the power to define and control women's reproductive and sexual resources.

Niddah and Mikveh in Contemporary Israeli Culture

When a woman has a discharge of blood which is her regular discharge from her body, she shall be in her impurity for seven days. —Leviticus 15:19

Israeli women are acquainted with a variety of beliefs regarding menstruation. The "modern" notion that menstruation is a normal, healthy, unmysterious physiological process is taught in family and sex education programs in Israeli schools. Contemporary folk culture has embraced such medicalized menstrual "syndromes" as PMS. Gynecologists are likely to treat menstruation as pathological if the menstrual cycle deviates from absolute regularity of timing or flow. Media advertisements for "feminine hygiene products" commodify menstruation. And traditional Jewish conceptualizations of menstrual purity and impurity continue to carry a great deal of weight for many women, even when juxtaposed to these other views.

Purity in Jewish culture is a multilayered, dense concept. Before the destruction of the Temple in Jerusalem in the year 70, the laws of niddah and mikveh were part of a sizable complex of laws dealing primarily with the Temple cult. With the destruction of the Temple most of these laws—with the exception of those concerning menstruation and childbirth—became irrelevant to Jewish life. As post-Temple Judaism developed, women's bodies became in a sense a symbol of the Temple, and some of the ritual and legal attention that had formerly been focused upon the Temple began to become focused upon women's bodies (see Meacham 1989). Over the centuries, preoccupation with women's purity became an expression of Jewish religiosity and identity (see Wasserfall 1992).

Jewish texts such as the Talmud and the Shulhan Aruch contain detailed exegeses of the Biblical law cited in the epigraph at the beginning of this section. Very briefly, couples are expected to refrain from sexual relations during the days of the woman's menstrual flow and for seven "clean" days afterward, following which the woman meticulously washes herself and then fully immerses three or more times in a ritual bath (mikveh) of "living water" (directly channeled rain water or spring water) in the presence of a mikveh attendant who has previously checked her to make sure that her body is truly clean. The couple is then allowed to resume sexual relations.[2]

For Jewish women, *halachic* (legal) treatment of menstruation is embedded within ideological conceptualizations that explicate and embellish the laws. For example, some Israeli women say that menstruation is a punishment given to women because of Eve's weakness or transgression. Linking menstruation (and its attendant cramps and "mess") with Eve draws the bodies of individual women into a mythic narrative, thereby imparting symbolic weight to women's physiological processes. By rooting menstruation in Eve's sin (her vulnerability to the snake which led her to endanger Adam), these women understand that they themselves suffer because of some essential female weakness. Part of the attraction of niddah and mikveh rituals is the opportunity to mitigate some of the consequences of Eve's punishment. Logically enough, some women perceive a connection between menstruation which removes blood from women in order make them pure, and the ritual salting that removes blood from meat in order to make it kosher (Cicurel 1998).

While only a minority of Israeli women (approximately one quarter)[3] attend the mikveh regularly, almost all Jewish Israeli women receive a "crash course" in mikveh ideology and practice when, as brides, they are obligated to immerse in the mikveh by the Orthodox rabbis who hold a monopoly on weddings and divorce in Israel. Outside of a few discrete populations of dedicated secularists,[4] most Israeli women are likely to have at least some contact with a friend, neighbor, relative, or co-worker who uses the mikveh and who extols its virtues. "Mikveh committees," active throughout the country, distribute literature on the mikveh and send out volunteers to teach women about the benefits of keeping the laws of ritual immersion. And at least among Israel's large North African and Asian ethnic populations, regular use of the mikveh never disappeared from the cultural map: Today's young women almost certainly have mothers or grandmothers who observed the laws of mikveh immersion. For these reasons, I see the conceptualizations and ritual routines of niddah and mikveh as constituting a corporeal landscape salient, or at least familiar, to the majority of Israeli women.

Mikvehs are located in almost every Israeli town and settlement, and in many neighborhoods in the larger cities. The Israeli mikveh establishment is quite institutionalized. Almost all mikvehs are administered by municipal religious councils; mikveh attendants are trained in courses run by state-sponsored rabbis; pamphlets and brochures available at the mikvehs are published by various governmental and nongovernmental agencies and organizations; and in some cities, such as Beer Sheva (see Cicurel 1998), the rabbinate employs women counselors who go door to door trying to convince women to use the mikveh and who organize meetings at which they teach about the benefits and laws of niddah. In the following discussion my own observations carried out over the past decade at mikvehs in Jerusalem are augmented by field work conducted by Inbal Cicurel in Beer Sheva and Ayelet Kaveh in Ramat Gan and Kfar Saba.

Israeli women frequent the mikveh for a number of reasons. For Orthodox and ultra-Orthodox Ashkenazi women, the mikveh is one aspect of a total lifestyle structured around observance of Jewish law. Most of the conversations that I held with ultra-Orthodox and Orthodox Ashkenazi women at the mikveh centered upon fine points of *halacha* (Jewish law) regarding timing of immersion (keeping track of the menstrual cycle and checking oneself internally twice each day during the week following menstruation to make sure that bleeding has ceased), worrying about having made a mistake of some sort regarding observance of the law (perhaps a bit of glue from an adhesive bandage had not been sufficiently removed from the skin, thus constituting a barrier between one's body and the water of the mikveh), fretting that the children at home have not yet been put to bed or that unexpected guests are wondering why the hostess has disappeared, or boasting about having managed to make it to the mikveh in difficult circumstances (as, for example, during a trip to Turkey, or when the extended family is visiting for a bar mitzvah, or despite having late meetings at work every night that week, and so on). These women were generally less than interested in long discussions (with me) about niddah and mikveh, and unless specifically asked rarely volunteered reasons for using the mikveh or feelings about keeping the laws of niddah.[5] If kept waiting in the communal waiting room, they usually read a book, crochet, or rest their eyes.

The other large category of mikveh attendees (in the 1990s) is comprised of second- and third-generation Israeli women whose parents or grandparents came from Asia or North Africa.[6] Most of these women consider themselves to be secular or traditional; a smaller number are Orthodox or ultra-Orthodox. The dress of the women in this group displays their fairly wide range of religious observance: Some wear skirts to below their knees while others come to the mikveh wearing sleeveless tops and shorts. Many do not observe other features of traditional Jewish law yet feel strongly about the importance of niddah and mikveh. The repertoire of reasons they offer for choosing to use the mikveh incorporates a range of personal, natural, and supernatural considerations. Some talk about the good feeling they have after immersing in the mikveh, a feeling of calm, spiritual uplifting, serenity, and total cleanliness of a magnitude that cannot be attained just from one's regular bathing and hygiene routine. Ayelet Kaveh's informants described "a feeling of dirt that has to come out [so you can feel clean], and clean from within" (26). Others speak about how you "feel brilliant, your face is radiant, shining." A number of women came to Kaveh after they immersed to show her the radiance of their faces. Especially interesting to me in these sorts of comments is the linkage of "spiritual" and "physical" dimensions. Women describe spiritual uplifting that occurs through bodily practices and bodily transformations that occur pursuant to spiritual rituals. What women are in fact portraying is a very particular construction of the female body—one in which women's physical state rather easily changes (for better or for worse) in response to their spiritual state. And conversely, spiritual rewards (and punishments) are meted out to women through their bodies.

The "Medical Basis" of the Niddah System

The Israeli mikveh establishment has developed rhetoric and techniques designed to draw women into mikveh observance. Although parts of the discourse generated by the mikveh establishment feel irrelevant to the secular and traditional Asian and North African women with whom I have spoken (for example, the rules concerning internal checking to make sure that bleeding has stopped), other aspects of this discourse resonate deeply and powerfully for many women, and have quickly become absorbed into the folk repertoire of beliefs about women's bodies.

One of the more popular mikveh booklets currently distributed to brides and made available at Israeli mikvehs is entitled *Nisu'in shel Osher—Happy Marriage* (Neriya 1989). Like other booklets of the same genre, it interweaves "expert" medical advice with Jewish law. The booklet "proves" the medical basis of the niddah system, opening with, "Dr. Shik Moyna, the researcher who became famous for discovering a test for diphtheria,[7] was the first to lecture in approximately 1920 on the topic of 'menstruants' poison—hemanotoxin'" (15). Afterward other "important professors" confirmed his findings, determining that menstrual blood contains a kind of poison that seems to damage men and fetuses, a fact "already known" to the medieval Jewish sage Maimonides. Weaving modern science and ancient misogynist taboos, the booklet continues: "It is customary to believe that this poison has a negative influence on materials that need to ferment, like yeast, dough, wine, and so on." In addition, "Most science recognizes another danger that threatens men who have contact with women during the niddah period. The menstrual discharge contains elements of blood, bits of the uterine wall, mucus, and various kinds of bacteria. When there is an open wound the bacteria can cause an infection [of the urethra]" (16). Women not only endanger men, but are even dangerous to themselves. "Medical science also recognizes the possibility that intimate relations during the menstrual period can damage the woman . . . There is a larger danger of infection in the pelvic area . . . It is accepted among specialists in gynecology that cervical cancer, a disease found among civilized and non-civilized nations, is rare among Jewish women who observe the laws of menstrual purity" (16). These scientific proclamations are interspersed with names of European physicians and esoteric bibliographic references, building an aura of incontrovertibly "expert" scientific proof.

The psychological aspects of menstruation are also addressed:

> It has recently been found that in women's bodies there is a temperature curve. From the day that menstruation starts until the middle of the cycle the temperature stays the same—low. Afterwards, it goes up and stays high until the day the next period starts. This cyclical movement marks all of the most important life processes for women—heart function, blood pressure, muscle strength, metabolism, etc. This movement also affects the woman psychologically. She has hours and days of uplifted spirits and loads of energy, which are switched by hours and days of the

opposite . . . Often, the woman's mood in the down days is low. In that period many women suffer from certain depression and from hypersensitivity. The feeling of discomfort leads to a desire to close oneself in and be alone. (18)

The booklet emphasizes that women are weak during the days of their period. Jewish law prohibits intimate relations for the seven days following menstruation, "the time in which the womb regains its strength. This also gives the woman a time for emotional calmness, and allows her to recover before resuming intimate relations." In Israeli mikveh discourse women's bodies are presented as so frail as to require a great deal of rest in order to carry out the tiring labor of sexual relations. In another booklet entitled *L'Bat Yisrael Likrat Nisu'eha—To the Daughter of Israel Approaching Marriage* (Neriya 1983), which is handed out to brides in a number of towns around the country, the young woman is advised to organize her month so as to do her heavy housework during the days in which she is forbidden to her husband, and in that way she can be more rested during the time when they can have sexual relations. On the day of her immersion she should sleep so she will be rested for the evening. "Sleep calms down the nerves and relaxes the muscles so that all of the organs are able to fill their task successfully."

Health and illness are central components of contemporary mikveh discourse in Israel.[8] Women are told—and tell each other—that sexual relations at the "wrong" time of month can cause cervical cancer. Mikveh booklets and counselors offer statistics showing that Jewish women have lower rates of cervical cancer, and quote doctors explaining that the uterus is more prone to infections which "may" cause cancer when it is "open" during menstruation and the week following menstruation. Inbal Cicurel has noted that in Beer Sheva the mikveh counselors explain to women that after menstruation a membrane starts to build up around the womb in order to protect a possible pregnancy. In the area of the vagina there is an acid that protects the womb from germs. The bleeding is alkaline and neutralizes that acid, and intercourse further jeopardizes the vulnerable womb. This folk medical model presents menstruation as a wound that takes seven days to heal, during which time the womb is vulnerable to germs. Over the course of the time in which she carried out her field work in Beer Sheva, Cicurel witnessed an increase in women offering medical explanations for keeping niddah and mikveh. As did Kaveh and I, Cicurel found that the source for these ideas is the mikveh establishment: books, mikveh attendants, counselors, and especially lectures by Orthodox gynecologists.

While it may be tempting to shrug off the idea that "You will get cancer if you don't dip" as an obvious rhetorical device used to convince women to observe the laws, it is important to understand that this rhetoric also constructs a certain kind of female body, a body that is naturally disease-ridden and requires "expert" guidance to avert disaster. According to Cicurel, the Beer Sheva counselors teach women that twice daily internal vaginal checks during the week following menstruation (to make sure that there is no further bleeding) is "preventative medicine" that may lead to early discovery of illness (cancer) and so save women's lives and especially their fertility. One wonders how women who indeed check themselves twice daily for at least one week each month (per rabbis' orders) are affected by holding the prospect of "discovering" malignancies so actively in their consciousness—whether they come to think of their bodies as always on the verge of being sick.

I make particular note here of the borrowing of a discourse propagated by the cancer establishment (oncologists, cancer associations, and so on). In current medical jargon early detection has been renamed "secondary prevention"—implying that submitting one's body to frequent expert examination can actually prevent cancer rather than merely reveal it at an earlier stage. While the borrowing of "preventative medicine" and "early detection" discourse seems to suggest a certain degree of cooperation between the medical and religious establishments, in this case the cooperation is more rhetorical than concrete. Despite the "preventative medicine" rhetoric, the rabbis who have authority over the mikvehs (at least in Jerusalem) have refused to allow women's health organizations to distribute or display material on breast self-examination at the mikvehs (although the timing of immersion after menstruation and the privacy afforded women during their extended bathing and other preparations for immersion make it a good opportunity for breast self-exam).[9] The rabbis claim that it will distract women from the "true" purpose of the mikveh.

Rabbis, mikveh attendants, and booklets such as *Nisu'in shel Osher* acknowledge the problems that can transpire if a woman's cycle is less than twenty-five days long, in which case ovulation occurs before immersion and the resumption of sexual relations, therefore hindering or even precluding conception. If this happens, according to *Nisu'in shel Osher*, the woman should go to a doctor who will give her hormones to "regulate" her menstrual cycle. In addition, she should take her temperature every morning to see when she ovulates. Acknowledging that ritual observances may exacerbate certain problems in women with short menstrual cycles, this advice construes ritually induced infertility as an illness appropriately treated by doctors. The suggested solution is for women to focus obsessive attention on their ovulation (in addition to the attention already focused on bleeding), to consult with a physician, and to take hormones (which may make them feel unwell or gain weight—a corporeal taboo of the highest degree for modern Israeli women). That many Israeli physicians collude in this practice, giving hormones to perfectly healthy women made "sick" by cultural codes, says a great deal about the cross-cutting ways in which various institutions work to construct female corporeality.

Mothers and Miracles at the Mikveh

Mikveh attendants hold a pivotal position in propagating mikveh ideology and in spreading miracle stories about the benefits of niddah and mikveh observance. While miraculous urban legends do take on a life of their own and circulate from mikveh to mikveh, the role of mikveh attendants in spreading the stories is crucial. The head attendant in a Ramat Gan mikveh is particularly fond of tales of infertile women who conceived after dipping in the mikveh. She, like other mikveh attendants, tells these stories replete with details and with individual twists: the problems faced by the particular infertile woman, previous attempts to conceive, the words the doctor used when he told her the good news that her pregnancy test had come back positive, and so on (Kaveh 1998).

The theme of fertility is central to mikveh discourse. We have seen that women's responsibility to bear children constitutes a meta-discourse in Israeli society. What we hear from mikveh attendants is a sub-discourse tying women's maternal duty to purity and obedience to Jewish law. A favorite story of the Ramat Gan mikveh attendant tells of a woman whose doctors discovered a large growth in her head. Before the operation to remove the growth, she came to the mikveh to dip and request God to take the cancerous grow from her head and put a live growth (a baby) in her stomach. Shortly afterward she discovered she was pregnant and went to the doctor to check the growth in her head. Miraculously, it was gone. This story, a fairly well-known Israeli urban legend, combines a number of motifs crucial to the cultural construction of women's bodies. First, the use of the same word, *gidul* (growth), for both cancer and fertility suggests that cancer and fertility are reversals of one another—analogous to other key dichotomies such as sickness and health, evil and good, and impurity and purity. Just as the transition from impurity to purity is mediated by ritual immersion in the mikveh, so is the transition from cancer to fertility. Pushing this symbolic construct a step further, I would suggest that the geographic transformation of the location of the growth from the "head" to the "stomach" further aligns purity and the national mission of motherhood with the body rather than with the mind or spirit; the good woman is one who embraces her corporeality and lets her stomach "grow"; the bad woman is one whose head "grows." A second motif intimates that in women purity and impurity—observance and non-observance of Jewish law—are manifested corporeally. Finally, this story revolves around the theme of authority over women's bodies. The heroine in the story submits to the authority of both God and the doctors. Religion and medicine are presented as simultaneously collaborating and competing for control of the woman's body; the doctor wants to operate but God cures her before the doctor has a chance to use his knife. In the end, the doctor is forced to admit his defeat when he tells the woman that the cancer has totally disappeared.

If sexual relations at the wrong time of month are injurious, dipping in the mikveh and keeping the laws of niddah are said to be healthy. Stories are told of women who suffered from a variety of diseases that were cured by dipping in the mikveh. The mikveh is also said to contribute to mental health and to happy marriages, and especially to fertility. Many stories circulate in Israel of relatives and friends who were blessed with children after they began properly to observe the laws of mikveh and niddah. Dipping in the mikveh in the ninth month of pregnancy is a well-known charm for an easy birth; dipping after a bride just emerged from the mikveh is a charm for conceiving.

Cicurel found the wish to protect husband and children to be the most frequently expressed explanation for keeping the laws of niddah separation. The women with whom she spoke translate *karet* (being "cut off" from the Jewish people—the Biblical punishment for sexual relations during menstruation) as any kind of accident to husband or children—from bike accidents to death. The Ramat Gan mikveh attendant, for example, tells of a little girl saved from falling from a high building because her mother dipped. I have often heard women say that observance of niddah and mikveh brings the woman's family one form or another of good fortune. Stories circulate about children or other family members who were saved from death or illness because the mother immersed in the mikveh. More generally, observance of menstrual rituals is said by women to have a positive influence on the family and household: to bring *sh'lom bayit* (conjugal harmony) and "make order in life." Women who began observing the laws of menstrual purity later on in their marriages often talk about the difference between "children of purity" and "children of niddah." Kaveh found that children "born in purity" were described as calm, serene, and responsible; the earlier children as more difficult to raise, stubborn, wild, and needing more parental supervision.

Perhaps the most poignant maternal mikveh stories have to do with a soldier who was saved because his mother dipped. Among the variants of this story are soldiers whose units were blown up but one soldier alone was saved, and soldiers who at the last minute were not assigned to units that were attacked by the enemy—both because the mothers dipped in the mikveh. Cicurel cites the story of a mother who inexplicably was urged by the mikveh attendant to pray for her family, beginning with her soldier son rather than with her seriously ill son. It turned out that the next day her soldier son was traveling with a group of fellow soldiers and their car fell off the side of a cliff into an abyss; her son was the only one to survive the accident.

The flip side of these stories, of course, is the understanding that mothers who do *not* dip endanger their soldier sons, a belief that fits well with the wider Israeli Jewish conceptualization of women as endangering the collective through the vulnerability of their demanding, female bodies. These stories seem to suggest that women protect and aid the state through corporeal rituals; that women's purity, together with men's fighting skills, defend Israel (see Yanay and Rapoport 1997). But whereas men perform specific actions to defend Israel, women's burden of defense rests inside their very bodies—a heavy load to carry, and one from which there is never weekend leave.[10]

Mikveh and Marriage

Contemporary mikveh discourse also emphasizes the effects of women's menstrual observances upon their marriages. Women who use the mikveh, mikveh attendants, and mikveh brochures concur that keeping the laws of niddah keeps the marriage fresh. I, like Cicurel and Kaveh, have heard repeatedly that mikveh observance will lessen the chances that your husband will cheat on you, get sick of you, or leave you. Among the advantages to observance of niddah cited most frequently by women throughout Israel is that it improves sexual relations with the husband. The enforced separation each month keeps one like "a bride all the time," it "preserves the excitement in marriage," and makes it "so the husband and wife won't get sick of each other" and will "continue to desire one another." Many women told me stories about straying men who came back to wives who began keeping niddah, or marriages on the verge of divorce that were saved when the wife's friend told her, "What do you have to lose, just try to go to the mikveh and it may help."

Cicurel interprets these sorts of marital anecdotes in terms of women's economic vulnerability and dependence upon men: Israeli society is highly consumer-oriented, yet women's salaries, significantly lower than men's, are rarely sufficient for attaining the standards of consumer achievement that women are encouraged to see as optimal. In the predominantly working-class Beer Sheva neighborhoods in which Cicurel carried out her field work, some women seem to view their immersion in the mikveh as a contribution that compensates for their lower contribution to family income. Cicurel, as did I, heard stories in which the observance of niddah protected a husband's job. A popular tale cited by Cicurel tells of a wife who started to observe niddah after a few years of marriage, and a few months later her husband told her of his new prosperity at work and asked her to keep on helping his business by continuing to immerse each month (n.d., 19). In a dramatically double-barreled variant on the theme of women's vulnerability, Cicurel has heard Beer Sheva mikveh counselors teach women that not observing the laws of niddah and mikveh may lead to cancer of the uterus, which leads to suffering and loss of fertility. But more than that, they also "tell the women that their husbands would not be able to carry the burden of a wife with cancer and thus by not keeping niddah, they may lose them as well" (10).

While contemporary mikveh discourse places a great deal of responsibility upon women and women's bodies—responsibility for the health, safety and prosperity of husband, children, and state—it is clear to women that authority in the matter of niddah and mikveh lies with men. Women are urged to consult with rabbis (or to ask their husbands to consult on their behalf) regarding a range of matters, including, for example, ambiguously colored vaginal secretions. Rahel Wasserfall itemizes the ways in which a husband can exercise control over his wife's mikveh observances: He can force her to have sexual relations before going to the mikveh, he can insist that she immerse before the completion of the seven "clean" days, and he can forget or refuse to send his wife to the mikveh (1990).

Brides and Menstrual Rituals

We turn now to a most particular type of female body, one that embodies and symbolizes not only the purity of the collective but also its very survival and continuity—the body of the bride.

Negotiations between Orthodox and secular political parties in contemporary Israel have bolstered a legal framework laid down by the Ottomans: The mainly secular state grants religious authorities exclusive jurisdiction over matters of marriage and divorce. This arrangement creates social inconsistencies that are problematic for women. In most spheres of public life, women are, by law if not always in practice, accorded the same rights as men. Women, like men, have the right to vote and to hold political office; women, like men, benefit from Israel's universal education and health care systems; Israeli law prohibits economic discrimination on the basis of gender. Israeli girls and women are told, in many arenas and in many ways, that they are full citizens of a democratic state and that they can expect equal treatment from the state and its institutions. Yet when women become engaged to marry—as most women do in Israel's pro-family and pro-natality culture—they encounter an entirely different understanding of gender and an entirely different set of social rules. In the framework of traditional Jewish practices and rituals of marriage and divorce, women and men are not equal.

This state-sponsored bifurcation echoes traditional rabbinic gender patterns. Talmudic scholar Judith Romney Wegner (1988) has argued that in the Mishnah and Talmud, Jewish women like Jewish men are considered to be people possessing both entitlements and obligations, and gender equality characterizes many spheres of life.[11] In the private domain of sexual and reproductive status, however, most women (including wives, minor daughters, and levirate widows) are considered legal chattel, who as property lacking rights and duties do not have jurisdiction over their own biological functions. Following Wegner's reading of the Mishnah and Talmud, it seems to me that the apparently inconsistent Israeli status quo (women can file complaints in labor court because of wage discrimination but must submit to an all-male rabbinic court in order to receive a *get* [bill of divorcement] that by Jewish law can be granted only by a husband and never by a wife) reiterates a very ancient and fundamental gender pattern already evident in the writings of the Sages.

As a consequence of the Israeli law requiring all weddings to be conducted by religious officials authorized by the state, Jews who marry in Israel are obliged to go along with a variety of ritual practices which, while often meaningless or even offensive to the bride and groom, are seen as religious commandments by the state-supported Orthodox religious establishment.[12] Perhaps the most intrusive practice is that requiring Jewish brides to immerse in the mikveh before the wedding, and to bring a note attesting to their ritual purity from the mikveh attendant to the rabbi who conducts the wedding. The obligatory prenuptial mikveh encounter—coming at a time of transition in personal and social identity in the lives of young women—exposes all Israeli women, not just orthodox women, to a persuasively presented, Jewishly "authentic," corporeal culture.

Before I turn to a more detailed discussion of ritual immersion of brides, I wish to make clear that the intense corporeal scrutiny during the mikveh ritual is but one part of a much broader construction of the body of the bride—the ultimate female body—as an object of legitimate public surveillance. Much of the traditional Jewish wedding sequence directs public attention to the bride's appearance. Perhaps the best example is the traditional Yemenite bride (in contemporary Israel a kind of iconic, folkloristic, collective bride) whose gown and headcovering weigh so much that she can hardly move. Unable to run, barely able to walk a few steps, her clothing makes her into a passive, visual platform for others to explore. Her dress and headgear are covered with myriad symbolic designs and objects embroidered and sewn onto the fabric. Yemenite folklorist

Zipporah Greenfield has spent twenty years studying a traditional Yemenite bridal dress; she told me it has taken her that long to "read" all of the symbols inscribed onto the body of the bride.

One of the still popular highlights of traditional Ashkenazi weddings is the *bedeken* ritual in which the groom walks up to the bride who is sitting passively and quietly on a queen's throne; he looks at her face for a moment, and then places her veil over her face. The collective, mythic meaning of the ritual is made explicit when the Biblical verses invoked for Rebecca before she was sent off to meet Isaac, her future husband, are pronounced: "O sister! May you grow into thousands of myriads. May your offspring seize the gates of their foes" (Genesis 24:60). The *bedeken* ritual dramatically assimilates the body of the bride to a mythic, national body. At some weddings the veil is opaque, literally blinding the bride; thus the bride indicates that "she is totally committed to her husband and has unquestioning trust in him" (Chill 1989, 280).[13] The palpable sexual charge of the *bedeken* ceremony (the bride and groom supposedly have not seen each other for some time before the wedding) hitches individual passion to legitimate sexuality to the future of the collectivity. The veiled bride bears on her body the textual legacy of Rebecca and the burden of (sightlessly) reproducing that legacy. Only the groom can uncover the face of the modest and pure bride; ownership is manifested as the right to reveal what is hidden from others.

In addition to these gendered corporeal constructions drawn from traditional Jewish scripts, the Israeli fashion industry—as is the case throughout the West—pitches beautiful and expensive gowns, hairstyling, and cosmetic applications for brides, items that accurately assume the bride's beauty to be an essential part of the marriage transaction and wedding ritual. Special salons for brides offer full-day treatments that include manicures, pedicures, depilation and waxing, facials, professional makeup, and hairstyling. This is typically followed by a round of photography shoots in front of culturally potent backdrops (famous buildings, shrines, gardens, and so on, visually associating the bride's body with national "treasures)."

In a pioneering study of how women's bodies are manipulated cross-culturally, Mary Daly (1978) has argued that rituals such as Indian suttee, Chinese footbinding, African genital mutilation, and certain aspects of Western gynecology dismantle the individual integrity of women; they function to prevent women from comprehending their own agency, from holding onto a sense of their own selves. By inscribing women's bodies with potent symbols, these sorts of ritual practices serve to trans*mute* real women into cultural icons and distance women from ownership of their own bodies. The wedding complex, and particularly the required mikveh immersion, seem to me to suit the model suggested by Daly.

Scrutiny of the young woman's body by a duly appointed representative of Jewish law and the Israeli state, and detailed instructions that prepare her to scrutinize her own body in preparation for subsequent monthly immersions, can be seen as techniques for teaching the bride—in a classic state of liminality—to view herself as a symbolic object rather than an autonomous subject. At the successful completion of the prenuptial immersion ritual, the mikveh attendant pronounces the bride a "pure daughter of Israel."[14] Several mikveh attendants told me how eager they are to use the opportunity of the compulsory prenuptial immersion to draw women into mikveh observance: the "nicest" room at the mikveh is always saved for brides, and attendants pride themselves on the time they spend talking to brides, a conversation that follows on earlier lessons by a mikveh counselor or rabbi's wife employed by the Ministry of Religion or municipal religious council.

Mikveh attendants, and the rabbis who direct their work, recognize that the prenuptial immersion presents a unique window of opportunity for drawing women into the niddah and mikveh system. Like officiants at rites of passage in other cultures, they understand that at times of transition the self is especially vulnerable and especially pliable. What surprises me is how quietly the non-Orthodox majority in Israel goes along with a ritual practice that involves repudiation of the bodily freedom and privacy of young women. While some brides find ways to trick or escape the mikveh system, few openly confront it; as far as I can ascertain, the compulsory immersion of brides has never been debated on the Knesset floor. One cannot but wonder whether the absence of public outcry reflects a certain acquiescence to a culture of gendered corporeal surveillance that, although not usually expressed through mikveh rituals by most secular Israelis, is in fact widely accepted as good and true. As we saw, much of the typical secular wedding sequence directs communal attention to women's passive bodies as well. Diverse streams in Israeli society, not only the Orthodox establishment, see women's bodies as potential sites of improper, impure, or dangerous behavior. The secular state, and not only the rabbis, institutionalizes through law its claim to a moral stake in women's bodies. Physicians and politicians join the religious establishment in justifying scrutiny of women's bodies and behavior through appeal to "higher" principles of the public good. And indeed, we have seen throughout this book that various institutions, not only the religious establishment, attribute heavy collective responsibility to women's bodies, while according women little authority or autonomy. Even the most secular Israeli brides, having recently completed their service in the IDF, are quite accustomed to "legitimate" institutional expressions of corporeal control.

Still, secular young women, raised on Western books, television, cinema, and educational curricula that (at least purportedly) teach independent thinking, are inclined to find the mikveh requirement burdensome. Brides may be made especially uncomfortable by the mikveh attendant who supervises the immersion, asking numerous questions regarding the date of the last menstrual period, whether during the seven days from the end of menstruation to the date of the ritual immersion the bride had twice each day inserted a cloth inside her vagina to check that the bleeding had stopped, and whether she had thoroughly cleaned her eyes, ears, nose, teeth, navel, hair, and so on prior to immersion.

Here is how one secular woman described her prenuptial mikveh encounter some years earlier:

> It was the most humiliating experience of my life. I felt like a baboon—when the mikveh attendant picked hair off my back [hair stuck on the body constitutes *hatsitsa*, a barrier between one's body and the water]. I felt like I was in a concentration camp. I felt like a baboon in a concentration camp.

This informant, I believe, did not use the words "concentration camp" lightly (these words are never used lightly in Israeli discourse); she used them to express her sense of the mikveh ritual as coercive and abusive. Still, as I said earlier, it is rare for brides to object openly to the mikveh requirement.

The anger of Israeli women is often directed at the mikveh attendant, who is felt to be "intrusive" by many brides, or who is perceived as holding the gates of the mikveh closed, for instance, to unmarried women who wish to use the mikveh. In fact, however, the entire system of niddah and mikveh is explicated by, arbitrated by, and controlled by male rabbinical authorities. The mikveh attendant is repeatedly told to make no decisions on her own, and a telephone for her to use to call the rabbi is one of the most essential pieces of mikveh equipment. Mikveh attendants hold heavy responsibility for the "kosher" (valid) purification of Jewish women—an error on their part could lead families into sin and have spiritual repercussions for the next generation. Yet they are told again and again by the rabbis who oversee the mikvehs that they must never make any *halachic* decision on their own, that they must call a rabbi even if the case at hand is identical to a case they saw the evening before (for example, a case in which a scab on a woman's body might constitute *hatsitsa* between her skin and the mikveh water, thus invalidating the immersion). The theme of responsibility without authority has, of course, surfaced throughout this book as one of the fundamental components of the Israeli cultural construction of women's bodies.

In addition to the mikveh immersion required by rabbis who officiate at wedding ceremonies, some Jewish ethnic groups in Israel continue to carry out traditional prenuptial mikveh ceremonies in which the family of the groom, represented by the groom's mother, plays a central role. The elderly Kurdish Jewish women among whom I have conducted field work in Jerusalem told me that it was a matter of principle for the bride's mother not to teach her about sexuality or niddah and mikveh, so that the bride would learn only the customs of her husband's family and not her own (Sered 1992). It is not uncommon nowadays to find that the mother-in-law competes with the mikveh attendant for the right to inspect, supervise, and control the bride's body.

The role of the mother-in-law is especially prominent at bridal mikveh parties. Parties at the mikveh were and still are celebrated the night before the wedding, particularly among North African Jews. At this occasion, women friends and relatives accompany the bride to the mikveh, where she disrobes and immerses in the ritual bath in the presence of her future mother-in-law and a small number of female relatives. While these parties do provide opportunities for groups of women to gather together away from the gaze of male authorities, and the singing and dancing that follow the bride's immersion are joyous and sometimes poke fun at men, the chief purpose of the parties is to provide the family of the groom with an opportunity to inspect the body of the young woman who will be entrusted to bear, birth, and raise their male descendants.

The groom's family has several interests that can be protected by the mother-in-law at the mikveh. First, they want to know that the bride is healthy and equipped with a normal female body; in other words, that she is a likely candidate for bearing healthy sons. Second, they want to know that the bride is not pregnant; in other words, that she will not pass off a child of another man into her husband's family. And third, the mother-in-law herself may want to test the waters and see that the bride is compliant; in other words, that she will accept the control of her mother-in-law and not behave as either a free agent or as a member of her natal family. The mother-in-law is delegated to organize relatives and guests, prepare food and music, and use the party to make a public statement that this bride is from now on part of her husband's family. Thus the mother-in-law, like the mikveh attendant, is a representative or a gatekeeper of a patriarchal institution in which she, as a woman, lacks full-fledged membership. Indeed, she herself was subjected to the same scrutiny when she was a bride.

An elderly Moroccan rabbi living in a Jerusalem neighborhood in which I have carried out field work (see Sered 1999b) talked to me about the meaning of traditional prenuptial mikveh rituals, opening with a discussion of henna (red dye spread on the hands of women throughout the Middle East, North Africa, and India at weddings and other ceremonies). Note his interpretation of the ritual as one in which symbols are literally stamped onto the body of the bride:

HeNnA stands for *Challa* [bread tithe], *Niddah* [laws of menstrual purity], *Hadlaka* [lighting Sabbath candles].[15] These are the three commandments that are necessary for the bride. I heard this from an official source. They teach the bride. They put the color on her hand so that she will look beautiful for the groom . . . They put it on her hand as a stamp [*hotemet*] that she has entered the correct Jewish life. It means that you have entered the burden of keeping the commandments.

Our conversation then turned to the issue of the presence of the mother-in-law when the bride immerses. Note here his explicit pronouncement regarding the ontological status of the bride: She is merchandise that is legitimately scrutinized and evaluated by potential purchasers and therefore she should not express agency, she should not "get angry."

It is written in the Mishnah [K'tubot 7:8] that they bring the relatives of the groom to check the bride, that she doesn't have any *moom* [defect]. It isn't her fault. Some kind of scar. Sometimes. They want to know and check the merchandise [*s'hora*]. We are not simple. Sometimes there is an argument. But if people understand the *halacha* [law], they take it in the correct spirit [that the law says the bride should be checked and rejected if she is sick or deformed]. This is an open eye. To see what is going on with the bride's body. The bride shouldn't get angry, it is written in the Mishnah to check the bride. The groom will see only her face before the wedding [not her entire body, so he can't know if she is normal and healthy].

The mikveh attendant's scrutiny of brides is an expression of the interest of the religious establishment (and of the state) in the bodies of women; the role of the mother-in-law is an expression of the interest of the extended family in the bodies of its women. These two sets of interests do not always sit well with one another and arguments are not uncommon when these two parties confront one another. Both sets of interests may also come into conflict with the perceived self-interest of the bride, shaped as it is by the Western entertainment industry with its marketing of romance and beauty and by the consumer economy with its emphasis upon female beauty (rather than upon purity, modesty, or fecundity). That brides tend to be more outspoken in protesting the intrusiveness of the mother-in-law than the intrusiveness of the mikveh attendant says a great deal about the relative powers of the state and of the family over women's bodies in Israel today. But more to the point, the conflict between the mother-in-law and the mikveh attendant rests on the shared assumption that women's bodies are legitimately controlled, that rituals enacted on women's bodies have implications for the collective, and that without the performance of corporeal rituals, women's bodies will be, in one way or another, impure, imperfect, and unhealthy.

Chapter 5

The Scrutinized Body

Under the Knife, in Front of the Camera, and in Back of the Bus

To My Sister—Do Not Feel Jealous.
There is nothing to be jealous of—you are worth more!
Don't be jealous of girls who go in immodest [*parutz*] clothing,
You are the modest ones—from you will come the continuation of the building of Israel.
You are the modest ones—in your merit Israel is holy and pure.
The Holy One Blessed Be He looks after you. And He hates hates hates the ones who go in immodest clothing.
There are men who do not manage to control their urges and look at those women who go around immodestly—Those women are the pathetic ones, they look for attention . . .
You should know—After men use immodest girls they throw them away like used toilet paper.
No man thinks of them seriously for marriage, for building a warm house with true and sincere love. With those girls it isn't love, just cheap and fleeting sexual desire.
And you, the modest and respectable one.
You—the kosher Jewish woman.
You are treated seriously like a woman of stature.
You will merit Gan Eden.
You will have the merit to bring righteous sons into the world.
You will have the merit to continue the generations of Israel.
You are the one whom the Holy One Blessed Be He admires and loves.
The woman who goes immodestly dressed inherits hell in the next world and in this world.
More than that, she shows to the public that she suffers from lack of attention and so she looks for attention from skirt-chasers in the street.
The woman who goes with a short skirt—she reveals the place of her stench, the place from which comes out stinking feces, stinking blood, stinking urine. And every place that the immodest one goes, she draws after her bad spirits, impure spirits, the spirit of prostitution.
So stay away from the company of ones like those. They are not suited to you. It is not your level. You, who wants holiness, must run away like from fire from women like that, so that they will not cause you trouble and destroy your house (for example, by stealing your beloved husband).
A question to think about: Why has disease increased in our generation? For example, uterine cancer, breast cancer, skin cancer, AIDS, foot pain?

Isn't it because of the immodesty of our generation?
And why are there more caesarian sections?
Isn't it a punishment for uncovering the stomach?
Remember: The length of the skirt must be at least 10 cm. below the knee.
In short: Dress and behave modestly and so save yourself from trouble and curse.
As a result of participating in and being present at mixed weddings, dancing, swimming, and these kinds of things, much sorrow and terrible things have happened: much adultery and prostitution, destruction of many good families, and especially sorrowful—masses of people, women, and children have been left broken, hurt, and miserable.

—Translation of a leaflet circulating in Israel in the 1990s, seemingly aimed at modern orthodox and traditional populations

Sanitas Hospital Celebrates Passover with an Unprecedented Sale

Breast augmentation: 12,100 shekels
Breast reduction: 14,800 shekels
And a free weekend for two in the Galilee!

—Advertisement appearing in Israeli newspapers, spring 1999

Throughout the day of July 14, 1998, a headline story on Israel's hourly government-run radio news broadcasts reported that a ministry of transportation driving tester had refused to test a woman whose clothing did not, to his sensitivities, sufficiently cover her body. News analysis shows were replete with discussions of exactly what the woman in question had worn. Dignitaries gravely debated whether the shirt had shown her navel or merely part of her midriff, her shoulders or only her upper arms. By that afternoon, Israel's central labor organization, the Histadrut, had crystallized its response to an incident that came to be construed as a conflict between the rights of government workers and the rights of women: Women have the right to dress according to their *taste*, but testers also have the right to refuse to test women according to their *conscience*. This particular incident was the only story concerning women broadcast that day on Israel's hourly news programs. Portrayals of women in the Israeli media frequently express concern with women's bodies: The message of newspapers, magazines, radio, and television is that women's bodies are interesting—women's bodies but not women's issues (women's issues are consistently superseded by security issues, which men, as current or former combatants or officers in the IDF, are believed to better comprehend).

Immediately following the news broadcasts of the driving test scandal, at least several times that day, listeners were treated to a particularly riveting commercial: An advertisement by Clinica On Medical Centers for the treatment of male sexual problems. The text of the advertisement went like this: "Where will your lawyer, your reserve duty officer, and your greengrocer NOT meet? At Clinica On." The rest of the ad boasted of Clinica On's private waiting rooms and separate entrances for its clients, in addition to the best urologists and sexologists with "full discretion."

These two items, broadcast one right after the other, both have to do with bodies in contemporary Israeli culture. Yet they reveal radically different treatments of men's and women's bodies. The discretion accorded men's bodies (and especially their sexuality) contrasts dramatically with the near constant and often public scrutiny of women's bodies (and especially their sexuality), a scrutiny so widespread that it is all but taken for granted.

In Israeli culture, scrutiny of women's bodies—with the possible exception of openly pornographic scrutiny—tends to be presented as a means to legitimate and noble ends. The most common expressions of corporeal scrutiny are linked to consumerism, fashion, advertising, and more generally Israel's increasingly capitalist ethos. As in other developed countries, Israeli newspapers and television are filled with photographs that invite the viewer to inspect women's bodies. And as in other developed countries, the merchandise advertised includes a range of products that claim to perfect women's corporeality, and an even larger range of products that are made attractive to the consumer through visual association with attractive women. This arena of public discourse is not unique to Israel, yet perhaps reaches new heights in Israel, where Pnina Rosenblum, voted "most typical Israeli woman" in a public poll, is a beauty queen *cum* glamour girl *cum* cosmetics industry magnate *cum* politician, and where teenage girls watch more hours per week of television than girls in any other European country (Harel, Kaneh, and Rahav 1997, 129).[1]

What is singularly Israeli is that the construction of the beautiful female consumer-consumable body coexists with deeply embedded, Jewish religious discourses of female corporeality. The consumer-driven scrutiny of women's bodies is mirrored in a religion-driven scrutiny, the most commonly specified reasons for which are modesty and purity—attributes considered especially important, yet especially precarious, in women.

Israeli women are watched by, and suffer corporeal harassment at the hands of, men who "admire" (that is, whistle, grab, make kissing noises at women passing by, and so on) and at the hands of men who "admonish." In both cases, public understandings tend to place the blame on the clothes worn by women; in both cases, public discourse presents the issue as one of (more or less reasonable) male response to women's clothing, rather than of direct and symbolic assaults on women's corporeal integrity. Women's bodies, in both cases, are understood to be, by nature, provocative targets of evaluatory gaze.

Unlike what is perhaps the dominant Israeli notion of maleness—the male body as quantifiable and thus "knowable"—female bodies are thought to be complex, capricious, and contestable, and thus legitimate objects for ongoing exercises in deciphering. In Jewish religious discourse, women seem to be defined as intrinsically immodest, a state that can be corrected only partially and temporarily through strict dress codes, continual supervision, and confinement to the domestic sphere. Because modesty and purity are understood to be precarious and impermanent states for women, "slippage," new demands, and friction are frequent. We shall see that a great deal of the public discourse regarding women's bodies has to do with acts of covering and uncovering. Through covering and uncovering, women's bodies are "read" for purity, modesty, beauty, wealth, and status —states that are never permanent. But more than that, the authority to cover or to uncover symbolizes power over the concealed or revealed body.

This chapter begins with a brief overview of secular constructions of female corporeality, concentrating upon the images promulgated by the mass media and advertising industries. These constructions are exemplified in the person of a woman who can be considered an icon of the consumer-consumable woman: Pnina Rosenblum, one of the sponsors of the Miss Israel competition.

In the second half of this chapter we shall see examples of the scrutiny of women's bodies in the context of accelerating Orthodox and ultra-Orthodox demands for female "modesty." The examples that I have chosen to analyze include the case of the Women of the Wall, several cases having to do with the dress of women government employees, several other cases concerning the presence of women in the public realm, and a few instances of enforced gender segregation in public places such as buses.

Although the demands made on women's bodies often sound as if they draw upon ancient, or at least highly traditional Jewish ideologies, it is crucial to understand that they are repeatedly created and recreated in a dialectical relationship with feminism, consumerism, and the modern capitalist economy. Religious fundamentalists in Israel, as in other societies, respond to feeling besieged and beset upon at the hands of a modern world (which seems to offer them few advantages) by vigilantly controlling the corporeal borders of their own community—that is, the borders of women's bodies (Douglas 1982). As global commerce brings a steady stream of new items into Israel's cultural repertoire, conflicts erupt over and over again. Put differently, the "temptation" of new possibilities for women and of changing fashions, cosmetics, and hairstyles elicits attention to women's bodies from a variety of religious and secular sources. What we will be looking at in this chapter, then, is not "simple" religious coercion, but rather expressions of institutional competition to define and control the cultural resource that is women's bodies.

Both media and religious portrayals of women present corporeal geographies of contestation that legitimate and encourage scrutiny, discussion, manipulation, and control—processes that augment the symbolic value of women's bodies at the expense of women's agency and autonomy. My goal in this chapter is to explore ways in which religious, political, and economic discourses construct the female body as a contested symbol, and I therefore want to clarify that what I am presenting are indeed processes; as cultural symbols, women's bodies are understood to be not static, but rather unpredictable and unreliable—in need of surveillance, investigation, and mending.

The Consumer-Consumable Body

The Media

Secular Israeli women, having rejected the modest and "pure" female corporeality of traditional Judaism yet having failed to attain the Zionist ideal of the brave warrior-farmer, find themselves inhabiting a corporeal void that the fashion, entertainment, and cosmetics industries are eager to fill. In contemporary Israeli culture, beauty and consumerism are gendered as female traits.

The presentation of women in the media both in the context of entertainment and in the context of consumerism (contexts that overlap a great deal) is similar to presentations in the United States: Successful women are sexually attractive, eternally young, and very slim. Anne Bolin has cogently argued that,

> What crosscuts the variety of female physiques is the linkage of beauty with femininity. Historically, Western somatic and sartorial ideals articulate with a culture of beauty . . . The culture of beauty chronicles the modification and mortification of the somatic self. It is intimately tied as a symbolic structure to fashion, adornment, dieting, and exercise and as an exonomic structure to capitalism. Women have come to be defined primarily in terms of allure and adornment, highly visible displays, and demonstrations of men's success. Capitalism and beauty conspire as a system in which seasonal changes in fashions as well as cycles in the female contour sell products. Women's ambivalence about body concept is institutionalized as a mechanism in the economics of beauty. (1992, 81–82)

Imbedded in the political economy of the cosmetics, fashion, and fitness industries, the unrealizable myth of beauty for women serves to suppress diversity, encourage depression and low self-esteem in women who believe that they do not meet elusive standards for presenting themselves and their bodies, and leads directly to a variety of health risks (for example, twenty-five years of evidence has shown that the chemicals used in manufacturing hair dyes cause cancers in animals [Zones 1997, 249, 268]).

Each year I am struck anew by the New Year's lists of "most newsworthy" Israelis that include men who "do" and women who are "seen" (or victimized). On one typical 1999 list of "top ten people in the news this year," the only women were Linor Abergil (the Miss Israel who was raped), Rena Resslan (the first Arab Miss Israel, whose photograph was being used to market a hair depilation company), and Shiran Franco (the nine-year-old girl who was rescued after being buried for four days and nights under the wreckage of a building in the Turkish earthquake). Of the men on the list six were politicians and one a top athlete.[2]

In an examination of 2,497 advertisements that appeared in Israeli daily newspapers and women's and men's magazines between 1979 and 1994, Anat First (1998) found parts of women's bodies used to highlight advertisement headlines, women displayed in various forms of subordination, men consistently appearing exaggeratedly taller than women, men portrayed engaging in some sort of activity while women tended to be portrayed in passive poses, and women more likely associated with cheap products and men with expensive and prestigious ones. According to First, by the mid-1990s gestures of subordination on the part of women were even more obvious than in the earlier pictures: Women were found more often on beds or floors (in physically "low" postures) or engaging in overt sexual behaviors. Bornstein and Ben-Ari (1997) looked at advertisements, published in the Israeli media in 1998. In more than half of the advertisements, women look to be in their teens, while only one-seventh of the men appear to be that young. Almost half of the women look seductive (photographed in sexually suggestive poses or with sexually inviting facial expressions such as puckered lips), while only one-fifth of the men do. And, more than half of the men appear to be satisfied in the picture's pose, whereas only one quarter of the women do. In sum, in advertising in the Israeli media (which both reflects and shapes the culture at large), women are eternally young, sexy, subordinate, and dissatisfied—not a particularly health-enhancing image.

Meirav Amram (1992) discovered a rather interesting Israeli twist on the "global" female advertisement form. Apparently, Israeli-made advertisements often show pictures of partially dressed or undressed women with their faces blurred or absent. Furthermore, in certain American and European advertisements adapted for the Israeli public, the woman model's face had been deleted.[3] According to Amram, the trend has been for clothed women to be photographed with clearly identifiable faces, and undressed women to be faceless. While I suspect that this convention is meant to protect the modesty of the young women shown in the advertisements, it also reinforces cultural conceptualizations of female bodies being somehow "more" bodily—these faceless, scantily clothed models represent utter, mindless corporeality. My favorite photograph of this genre is an advertisement brochure for an exhibit of products and information for mothers and pregnant women. The photograph on the cover of the brochure displays three pregnant abdomens—three faceless, mindless, and legless wombs.[4]

I am especially intrigued with instances of juxtaposition of traditional Jewish imagery or customs and modern commercialism. "Sanitas Hospital Celebrates Passover with an Unprecedented Sale," declares one 1999 advertisement in large and eye-catching letters. The naïve reader who expected to learn of a sale on specially healthful matzah crackers or ceremonial wine would have been disappointed. The 1999 Passover celebration sale was for "breast augmentation: 12,100 shekels [about $3,000]; breast reduction: 14,800 [about $3,500] plus a weekend for two free in the Galilee."[5] And advertisements of this sort do seem to work. According to an article in *HaAretz* (August 30, 1999) the number of breast enlargement operations in Israel has risen by 250% in the last two years.[6]

As in other Western countries, violence against women is sometimes hinted at and sometimes made explicit in Israeli advertisements. One advertisement shows a woman in sexy underwear blindfolded and tied to a chair: "We had to tie this girl up, because she grabbed at the [Pesach] Holiday sales" (an ad for Only Jeans). But the ad that I have found most memorable consists of a full page, most of which is left blank. A large, sharp knife is drawn diagonally across the top of the page. The text of the ad reads: "Plastic surgery is not something you buy *'al ha-sakin*" (literally, "on the knife"), an expression that usually refers to a vendor opening a watermelon with a knife so that the purchaser can see that it is red and ripe inside. The rest of the ad addresses a female audience; every "you" that follows is in the feminine: "Have you dreamed of plastic surgery that will make you beautiful, that will change your life? Have you heard of inexpensive surgery—and were conned into it? But you paid a big price for it: the surgery failed and could not be reversed, and the dream turned into a nightmare." The ad then claims that their clinic never does such things. The bottom half of the page shows four very busty women. This ad, visually associating women, victimization, and violence, is well designed to cash in on Israeli fears of knife-wielding terrorists out to brutalize "our" beautiful and sexy women.

"The Rosenblum"

Pnina Rosenblum is the national icon of secular female corporeality. Over the past two decades she has been called "the most typical Israeli woman," "the Israeli princess," "Israel's best-known sex symbol," "the Israeli Barbie

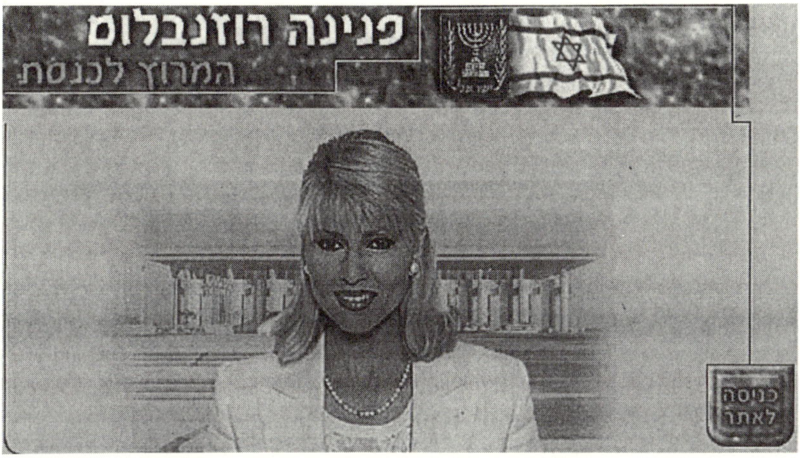

Pnina Rosenblum standing in the front of the Knesset, with the flag and seal of the State of Israel overhead. The background is colored in Pnina's trademark pink. The caption reads "I thank you for visiting the site of the Pnina Rosenblum Party, led by Pnina Posenblum."

doll," and "the breasts of the nation." In the course of her career, she has made the transformation from consumable (beauty queen) to consumer (glamour girl) to consumption magnate (president of her own cosmetics company) to politician touting a vague platform of women's rights.

Pnina Rosenblum first came to public notice when she won a series of beauty contests as a teenager. This stage of her career culminated in being crowned Miss Israel. In the wake of her success, she held a number of jobs that capitalized on her physical appearance; at one point she worked promoting an appliance to improve breast tone. Following a number of years in which she lived abroad as a golden glamour girl,[7] Rosenblum returned to Israel and parlayed her beauty contest fame into a lucrative cosmetics company. Unlike most other cosmetics company magnates who have to hire beautiful women to entice customers, Rosenblum sells her products by selling herself. In an interview published in the *Wall Street Journal* (August 14, 1992) on the occasion of her company's becoming the fastest growing cosmetics business in Israel, Rosenblum commented, "I know what women want. They want to look like Pnina Rosenblum." In 1998 Rosenblum announced the founding of the Pnina Rosenblum Party (later changed to *T'nufa* [Momentum]) and ran (unsuccessfully) for the Knesset in the 1999 elections. Even as the founder of a party, Rosenblum sold her platform by selling herself. Her message to the public was: Look at me, I came from an impoverished home and I succeeded, and you can too.[8]

Feminist and women's organizations have not been enthusiastic about Rosenblum's political bid, primarily because she does not have a feminist track record. The chair of the Israel Women's Network commented that, "It seems that the media and the public have concentrated on the body of Pnina instead of on the body of the issue. Her pictures show up everywhere, while the issue of guaranteeing representation of women in the Knesset and the government melted away" (*HaAretz*, March 2, 1998; byline Meirav Sari Vervitras). Still, many Israeli women like Pnina's brand of feminism. In a survey conducted by the women's magazine *LaIsha* in February 1999, readers were asked who most embodies their idea of the successful woman; 42.8% chose Pnina Rosenblum, while only 9% chose Limor Livnat (Likud Party), 2% Shulamit Aloni (Meretz Party), and 1.3% Yael Dayan (Labor Party). In a poll conducted by Gallup for *Ma'ariv*, Rosenblum was chosen in the top ten of admired Israelis, together with Yitzhak Rabin, Shimon Peres, Benjamin Netanyahu, Menahem Begin, Ezer Weizman, David Ben-Gurion, Ariel Sharon, Amnon Lipkin-Shahak, and Rita (a popular singer, and the only other woman to make it onto the list) (*Yedioth Aharonoth*, *7 Yamim*, July 31, 1998; byline Einat Berkovitch).

Orna Coussin in *HaAretz* writes that Pnina Rosenblum is

> a label, a generic name, like Hoover or Pelephone. How many times have we seen her name in the newspapers without any title at all? Not "businesswoman Pnina Rosenblum," nor "cosmetics company owner, Pnina Rosenblum," but just plain Pnina Rosenblum. Sometimes the name refers not to Rosenblum but to what she represents, the prototype of a certain kind of woman. There are women who "want to be Pnina Rosenblum" or who "dress like Pnina Rosenblum." (March 9, 1998)

As I collected material on Pnina Rosenblum I noticed that in newspaper and magazine articles she often is referred to as "The Rosenblum" (*HaRosenblum*), transforming her name from a proper noun to a generic one—making her a symbol, an icon, rather than an individual.

In the course of a lengthy interview, which included visits to Rosenblum's house and office, reporter Einat Berkovitch observed the many pictures of Rosenblum hanging on her walls, and the way in which Rosenblum related to the pictures. Intermittently walking over to photographs of herself, Rosenblum repeatedly made comments such as, "What a wonderful smile I have," "My waist is amazing, isn't it?" and "That hairstyle that I had, the one the whole country copied." A great deal of conversation was devoted to her physical appearance: how thin she is, how beautiful she is, how well she is made up (*Yedioth Aharonoth*, *7 Yamim*, July 31, 1998). Especially striking in Berkovitch's report is the extent to which Rosenblum views herself as an object to be scrutinized. Rosenblum is indeed a success story: She has learned to see her own body through the gaze of the fashion and beauty industry.

Ironically, while Rosenblum is invariably characterized in the press as "blonde" (no matter what the topic of the article), she is forthcoming about the fact that her natural hair color (brown) is insufficient and that she dyes her trademark platinum hair. As an icon for women to emulate, Rosenblum embodies the body that "needs work."

In an Independence Day interview pursuant to having been voted the "typical Israeli woman" in a public poll, Rosenblum explained that this title is appropriate because she is an embodiment of the nation. "Everything that happens here excites me personally. If something bad happens, right away I become agitated." Even during the five years she lived in London and New York she would defend Israel in discussions and arguments. "I remember once in a casino in London I argued so much with a Palestinian that I got a stomach ache from nerves and they took me to the hospital." While hardly suggesting that every word uttered by Rosenblum be treated as holy writ, I am struck both by her self-portrayal as the "ideal" or "typical" woman who becomes sick defending her country, and by the newspaper's decision to publish that seemingly trivial bit of Rosenblum's interview (*Yedioth Aharonoth*, April 13, 1994).

Press reports reinforce Rosenblum's inclination to explain her business and political career in terms of her bodily history. The press repeats the fact that Rosenblum was unable to have children of her own and so adopted two children, and thus her political party advocates universal access to fertility treatment and easing of adoption procedures. Repeated media references to Rosenblum's infertility suggest that even the "breasts of the nation" does not have a good enough body. Repeated references to her history of infertility may also be seen as hinting at cultural discomfort with a woman embodying both successful fertility and successful sexuality: One or the other is quite enough (and each is a significant social resource), but put together under the control of a strong woman, they threaten the patriarchal order.

In late December 1998, an interview with Pnina Rosenblum appeared in papers throughout the world in an Associated Press story by Lauri Copans. The headline set out the symbolic framework of gendered Israeli politics: "IN A GENERALS' RACE, A BEAUTY QUEEN THROWS IN HER CHAPEAU." Copans wrote,

> One political outsider kept her uniform on when she jumped into Israel's political fray. In an election campaign increasingly dominated by former generals, former beauty queen Pnina Rosenblum provided a fresh face. Well, a heavily made-up face. The former Miss Israel markets a popular line of cosmetics in Israel, and didn't lack for her creations when she ventured into the Jerusalem streets Thursday. "What a beauty," exclaimed one fan, hugging Rosenblum at a mall. "I washed my hair with your shampoo this morning."

Copans compared the political emergence of recently retired Chief of Joint Staff, Lieutenant General Amnon Lipkin-Shahak, "who doffed his uniform for civilian clothes Thursday," with Rosenblum, who "was in full battle dress: form-fitting Pnina Rosenblum black suit, miniskirt hovering over sheer black Pnina Rosenblum stockings."

Polls conducted in the months before the May 1999 election consistently showed Pnina Rosenblum's party winning one or two seats in the Knesset. In a study funded by the Israel Women's Network in late 1998, 8% of women and 2% of men polled said they were planning to vote for Rosenblum's party, and another 13% of women and 7.5% of men said they were considering it. Yet in a pattern that we have seen repeatedly throughout this book, Rosenblum's corporeal accomplishments did not translate into political power: Her party did not receive enough votes for even one seat in the Knesset. Even a supermodel does not have the power of a general; earrings and guns are not equal corporeal decorations.

A bundle of symbolic inversions, Pnina Rosenblum is the "breasts of the nation" who cannot bear children; she is the "blonde bombshell" who has to dye her hair; she is Miss Israel whose party does not garner even one seat in the Knesset; she is a flamboyant individual who has become a generic name. "HaRosenblum" symbolizes the possibility of a woman succeeding by her wits and strength of character, and she symbolizes the impossibly slim, youthful, blonde, glamorous beauty that drives young women to anorexia and older women to cosmetic surgery.

Women, Ritual, and the Orthodox Gaze

Rights/Rites of Baring/Bearing Arms

Amidst illustrated interviews with Pnina Rosenblum and advertisements for diet regimes and cosmetic surgery, the series of incidents and controversies described in the following pages appeared in mainstream, secular Israeli newspapers of the past decade. Although many of the stories involve ultra-Orthodox individuals, groups, or leaders, all have become part of a much wider Israeli discourse. The diffusion of gendered religious conceptualizations occurs for a number of reasons and in a number of ways: Official state recognition and monetary backing are given to religious institutions such as the Chief Rabbinate and municipal religious councils; ultra-Orthodox groups and individuals make demands that directly affect the bodies of secular women; the tendency to treat ultra-Orthodox Jews as icons who embody the traditional Jewish past imbues rabbinic pronouncements with a certain halo of holiness that continues to influence large portions of the Israeli population; and the secular press frequently channels stories from the ultra-Orthodox community out into the larger secular world.

In an exceptionally insightful headline, the *Jerusalem Post* of August 9, 1996, declared: "THE ULTRA-ORTHODOX ATTEMPT TO CONTROL JERUSALEM IS BEING WAGED OVER THE BODIES OF LOCAL WOMEN." The text of the article reported a series of verbal, spitting, and rock-throwing attacks on women Ministry of Education employees at a ministry branch located on the seam between downtown Jerusalem and the ultra-Orthodox Mea She'arim neighborhood. Apparently, the clothing practices of the ministry's employees did not meet ultra-Orthodox standards for women's modesty. During the six weeks preceding the newspaper report, more than thirty women had been attacked in the neighborhood of the ministry, and ministry women had staged at least one protest demonstration.

According to a report in *HaAretz* (August 7, 1996), Ministry of Education women had urine poured on them when they parked near their office. One woman employee testified that she herself had been attacked when wearing "a calf-length skirt and a loose T-shirt with a crew neck and elbow-length sleeves." A story in *Ma'ariv* (July 30, 1996) reported that while parking her car near the ministry, Sigalit Omer, a ministry employee, was surrounded by a gang of ultra-Orthodox men who rocked her car side to side, threw eggs at it, hit it with metal pipes, and said they would kill her. Her rescue came in a form surprisingly standard in cases of the sort: She was saved by two Arab workers who saw the attack.

The press reported that an undercover policewoman sent to the neighborhood of the Ministry of Education as a decoy (she was instructed to wear a sleeveless dress and walk around in the neighborhood) was violently assaulted. Upon leaving the car, "I heard a man shouting, 'Whore, get out of here.'" As we shall see, this kind of derogatory sexual language is typical in gendered confrontations. Two hours later, when she returned to the car another ultra-Orthodox man shouted the same epithet, and then picked up "a large rock" and threw it at her. As the police waiting nearby arrested the assailant, an ultra-Orthodox woman "came closer to me, screamed all kinds of curses and hit me hard" (*Jerusalem Post*, August 9, 1996).

Deputy mayor of Jerusalem Haim Miller (a representative of the ultra-Orthodox Yahadut HaTorah Party) demanded that the Ministry of Education instruct its employees to come in suitable clothing to work "and not like to the sea shore" (*HaAretz*, July 31, 1996). Miller's comments invoke two somewhat distinct issues: The first concerns *who* has the right to determine what women should wear, the second shifts the focus of the conversation away from who to what—what style of clothing is appropriate. This double-pronged rhetorical approach draws attention away from the more significant issue of corporeal authority: In a culture accustomed to gazing at women's bodies, discussions of "what she was wearing" easily overshadow the deeper question of who controls women's bodies.

HaAretz (July 31, 1996) reported that posters had gone up around the neighborhood of Mea She'arim demanding that the offices of the Ministry of Education be moved from "our neighborhood." The posters, invoking a language of purity ("our camp [*mahaneinu*] will remain pure"), called on ultra-Orthodox residents to prepare themselves for a struggle. Mea She'arim men framed their objection to the "immodest" clothing of the ministry women in culturally resonant terms: "They [the women] *pollute* [*m'tam'ot*] the eyes of our children" (*Ma'ariv*, September 30, 1996; my emphasis). This short sentence attributes cosmic, or at least symbolic, danger to women's bodies. The danger inherent in women's bodies, it seems, is specifically menacing to children; women's bodies in their "natural" state imperil the collectivity's future.

The response of government officials to the harassment of ministry women was neither swift nor severe. Jerusalem Mayor Ehud Olmert and Education Minister Zebulun Hammer remained conspicuously silent. Benzion Dell, the ministry's director-general, issued a statement on July 30, 1996, that condemned an attack on one particular worker, suggesting that the attack was perpetrated by "delinquents" and expressing hope that "those in charge of maintaining law and order" would respond appropriately. His response reduced systematic attacks on women to an attack on one woman by "delinquents." Dell's senior assistant, Michael Cohen, explained to the press that the Ministry of Education compound does not have room for all of the workers' cars, and tenured workers have priority for the parking spaces. He added, "They [women] don't have to park there [in the lot behind the ministry, where some attacks have occurred]. They could park somewhere else." Cohen's remarks both ignored that attacks had occurred all over the neighborhood, and insidiously injected the well-known "blame the victim" refrain. Pouring salt on wounds, Cohen implicitly reminded his audience that few women reach senior tenured ranks, even in a government department in which most of the employees (teachers and clerks) are women.

In August 1996, in the wake of dozens of assaults, a demonstration was held in the Ministry of Education courtyard (*Jerusalem Post*, August 7, 1996). With the exception of ministry employees who testified to having been personally assaulted, the orators' rhetoric centered on religious coercion as a political issue, and made little direct reference to attacks on women *qua* women. Instead of framing the attacks as assaults on women's bodies, public discourse has tended to frame the attacks as part of a "larger" battle in which women's bodies are "merely" the battlefield. Thus, the press (*Yerushalayim*, August 2, 1996) reported on a meeting between leaders of the ultra-Orthodox religious court and the deputy commissioner of police for the Jerusalem district at police headquarters. At that meeting the ultra-Orthodox leaders suggested a deal: They would put up posters calling on their community to stop the violence and rock throwing at ministry women if the police would release from jail a number of ultra-Orthodox men who had been arrested at other recent demonstrations.

A new set of signs addressed to secular women has been put up recently in ultra-Orthodox neighborhoods. These signs proclaim that "Parking and passing through [this neighborhood] in immodest clothing is absolutely forbidden. We are not responsible for damage caused to those who disobey. You have been warned." The not-so-covert threat of violence in the wording on these signs is part of the spiraling war over women's bodies of which the Ministry of Education attacks are but one episode. The threatening wording of these signs implies, of course, that "immodestly" dressed women bring violence upon themselves, a claim identical to the old and vicious claim that men are driven to rape by the seductive clothing of their victims.

The Jerusalem newspaper *Kol HaIr* (July 12, 1996) reported an incident in which a woman "wearing a miniskirt" suffered a bucket of dirty water poured on her head from a balcony as she walked along a main street in downtown Jerusalem. People watching from a bus station across the street said they had seen another woman treated in the same way a few days earlier. When the woman went to the police to complain, the officers on duty immediately knew at what address this had happened, suggesting that she was not the first to complain. Still, at least up through the time of the newspaper investigation, the police had not taken any action. What I draw attention to in this report (published in a notoriously secular newspaper) is the press's acceptance of the rules of the game: The woman's clothing (miniskirt) is presented in the article as the immediate cause of ongoing acts of abuse and violence. Reports of this sort draw the woman victim into the story as complicit (after all, she wore a miniskirt), and frame her choice of clothing as a legitimate matter for public scrutiny.

In a number of the incidents reported in the press, ultra-Orthodox women assaulted and tried to tear the clothing off of secular women who ventured into ultra-Orthodox neighborhoods. *Ma'ariv* (May 13, 1997), for example, ran a picture of an enraged-looking ultra-Orthodox woman ripping at the dress of a secular woman filmmaker. The incident took place in the Armenian Quarter of the Old City of Jerusalem on a Sabbath when a film crew (which had received permission from neighborhood residents) came to shoot their movie. Soon after arriving, they were attacked by two ultra-Orthodox women, who spit at them, cursed them, kicked them, threw cans at them, and tried to pull off the clothes of the women crew members, stopping only when a couple of Arab men working nearby intervened. (It seems to me that pulling off women's clothes is a means of "exposing" them for what they are—harlots and sluts. The Women of the Wall have similarly had their haircoverings pulled off by ultra-Orthodox women, as we shall see). According to reports, police saw the attack but did not arrest the attackers because the ultra-Orthodox women were not willing to go into the police car on the Sabbath. (The police summoned them to the station later that week, but they did not show up.)

A headline in *Ma'ariv* quoted one of the attacked women: "The ultra-Orthodox attacked us and Muslims came to our defense. I understood who my real enemies are." The theme of Arab men who save secular Jewish women from violent attacks by religious men and women has appeared a number of times in public discourse over the past decade. While we could read these reports as simple factual accounts, the press clearly has a great deal of leeway in choosing what details to report and how much weight to give various details. In the case of the film crew, the Arab saviors of secular women were placed in the headline. I suspect that this thematic scenario is so compelling because it hints at the unexpected: The "expected" scenario is one in which Jewish men (soldiers) protect Jewish "womenandchildren." The image of Arab men protecting a Jewish woman—in this case from another Jewish woman who is trying forcibly to undress her—tickles (titillates) the public fancy.

One well-publicized incident in which women's bodies and voices elicited controversy occurred during the planning for President Ezer Weizman's swearing-in ceremony in 1998 for his second term of office. The ceremony was to take place at the Knesset, and women soldiers along with men soldiers were scheduled to sing. Certain ultra-Orthodox Knesset members objected to the audible presence of the women, saying that they would be "forced" to leave the Knesset hall if women sang. When President Weizman was informed that Knesset policy had been to allow only male performers, it was decided to invite the male soldiers from the original troupe, but not the female soldiers (*Ma'ariv*, May 13, 1998). Using the language of male "sensitivity" (which typically is presented as standing in contrast to female "taste"), it was reported that while the IDF was not actively involved in making this decision, it was done to "avoid offending the *sensibilities* of religious Knesset members" (*Jerusalem Post*, May 13, 1998; my emphasis). After several days of heated opinions voiced in the press, President Weizman decided to opt out of the conflict by canceling the Knesset performance entirely. Throughout the episode, women's bodies and voices were treated as symbols for a variety of political issues; the real women involved were lost in the contentious debates. Thus the left-wing political party Meretz made a public statement that, "This is another expression of the efforts of the ultra-Orthodox to take over our lives." (In the 1999 Knesset elections the first three slots on the Meretz list were held by men, and the two Meretz members appointed to sit in Barak's cabinet were both men,[9] so it is not quite clear to whose lives Meretz's "our lives" referred.) Avraham Poraz from the liberal Shinui party called the incident "religious coercion of artists in Israel," somehow missing the fact that coercion was aimed only at the bodies of women. Knesset member Yael Dayan (Labor) was one of few politicians to have understood (or to have admitted to understanding) the gendered and institutional stakes. Dayan commented to the press that, "They kicked out women (*he'ifu nashim*) just because they are women. If this were a civilian group, the women would not have agreed to this. But here they are prevented [from objecting] because they are soldiers receiving an order" (*Ma'ariv*, May 14, 1998). What Dayan pointed to is the complexity of the contestation; the issue was not simply "secular versus religious" or "artistic freedom," but rather several powerful institutions (the presidency, the Knesset, the IDF, and the religious establishment), all of which command significant resources, competing to control that double-loaded symbolic resource—the "woman soldier."

Women in Black and Women of the Wall

Our next example deals with modesty not in the narrow sense of covered knees and elbows, but rather in broader Jewish cultural meanings of "appropriate" gendered corporeality. We shall see a group of women, striving to define themselves as intellectual and spiritual activists, vociferously reminded of their sexual and reproductive identity.

The Western Wall, a remnant of the Jerusalem Temple complex that was destroyed almost two thousand years ago, is commonly believed by Jews to be the holiest place on earth. Before the destruction of the Temple, the priestly cult was centered there. Still today, written petitions to God are placed between the cracks of the stone wall, implying that God is in some way especially present at the Wall. The Wall is today not only a religious symbol but also a national and military one. Film footage of the recapture of the Wall during the Six Day War is often shown on television, and each year the IDF Paratroopers induct new (male) soldiers into their ranks at a dramatic ceremony held at the Wall. The paved area in front of the Western Wall is divided by a barrier separating the men's section from the women's section, as is customary in Orthodox synagogues. On the men's side one finds individual men praying, and *minyanim* (prayer quorums comprised of ten adult men) engaged in vocal communal worship. On the women's side one sees only individual women praying. This is in keeping with traditional Jewish notions of men as constituting the public community and women remaining private individuals—a gender configuration that constitutes a geography of power (decisions that affect the community as a whole are made in the public realm). In a revealing case of politics making strange bedfellows, the IDF seems to go along with Orthodox insistence on privileging male access to the Wall. According to the newspapers, as of February 1993, women choirs and recordings of women choirs would no longer be allowed to take part in IDF ceremonies at the Wall, a policy agreed upon by IDF Chief Rabbi Major General Gad Navon, Rabbi Yehuda Getz, and the IDF officer responsible for the ceremonies (see *Jerusalem Post*, November 18, 1993).

The story of the group of women who came to be known as the Women of the Wall began on December 2, 1988, when a gathering of approximately one hundred women participants in the First International Jewish Feminist Conference in Jerusalem held a prayer service at the Western Wall. American-born women for the most part, they were accustomed to the more egalitarian religious modes that characterize American Judaism. They went to the Wall holding a Torah scroll (traditionally read only by men), several of the women wearing *tallitot* (prayer shawls traditionally worn only by men), and many wearing *kippot* (skullcaps, also traditionally worn only by men). The group entered the women's section and proceeded to conduct a communal prayer service. The response was violent; other women praying in the women's section and men praying in the men's section attacked the women both verbally and physically. The women pledged to return to the Wall on the first day of each month to carry out their prayer services. Following a series of assaults, they sought a court order demanding, among other things, that the police offer them protection. This case has been in and out of the Israeli courts and government committees for ten years, with no resolution in sight.

While the main combatants in this episode have been the Women of the Wall and the religious establishment (including the Ministry of Religion, the rabbi with jurisdiction over the Western Wall, and the Israeli chief rabbis), secular newspaper reporters and editors and other public figures have also had their say, which has not been consistently sympathetic to the Women of the Wall (see Kampf 1996), who are seen as American "Reform" interlopers trying to appropriate a state symbol of national (not only religious) identity.[10]

I have traced the story of the Women of the Wall in detail elsewhere (Sered 1997b). What interests me here is the rhetoric that has been used by those who oppose the Women's presence at the Wall. In the discourse of their adversaries, it is difficult to distinguish between the demonization of women's bodies as an end in itself, and the demonization of women's bodies as a means to accomplish other aims (in this case, ultra-Orthodox control of a valued national holy site). For example, the *New York Times* of February 12, 1988, quoted Rabbi Getz (the State-appointed rabbi who has jurisdiction over the Western Wall) as saying, "A woman carrying a Torah is like a pig at the Wailing Wall." This kind of comment is not lightly made. Pigs, in the Jewish cultural imagination, are far more than a forbidden variety of meat. Pigs symbolize all that is polluted and un-Jewish. In Rabbi Getz's words, the Women's presence at the Wall constitutes a symbolic threat to collective purity and identity. And indeed, the insults shouted at the Women by other men and women at the Wall are telling: pigs, polluted (*tame'*), gentiles (*goyim*).

"Prostitute" is one of the more common profanities shouted at the Women of the Wall. *Yedioth Aharonoth* (March 21, 1989), for example, reported that ultra-Orthodox women screamed at the Women, "Nazis, go to monasteries and have Christian babies there!" Both in their legal briefs and in their efforts to calmly explain their presence to others at the Wall, the Women evoke Jewish law and have become expert in its intricacies in matters of women and liturgy. Yet while the Women of the Wall labor to argue rationally from within the Jewish legal system, their assailants (both in court and during the sometimes violent confrontations at the Wall) refuse to enter into legal discussion with them at all, instead reminding them that despite their desire to constitute a spiritual group they remain grounded in corporeality—"prostitutes." Tirades concerning women's bodies have even been shouted at women politicians who came to the Wall to investigate the situation. For instance, ultra-Orthodox Jews yelled "Arafat's prostitute" at Knesset member Yael Dayan when she toured the Wall site together with Knesset members Anat Maor and Naomi Hazan (*Ma'ariv*, November 11, 1996).

The central place of bodily discourse in the conflict of the Wall is brought home in a headline to an opinion piece written by Israel Eichler, a self-styled spokesman of the Jerusalem ultra-Orthodox community: NO ONE PREVENTS ANYONE ELSE FROM PRAYING AT THE WALL IN HIS [*sic*] OWN FASHION. BUT THE WALL IS THE LAST PLACE TO CARRY OUT A BATTLE FOR THE RIGHT OF A WOMAN TO WEAR A TALLIT, READ FROM THE TORAH, WEAR A KIPPA, AND GROW A BEARD. Through his efforts to naturalize religious gender roles via reference to the body (a woman reading from a Torah is like a woman growing a beard), Eichler's proclamation reveals the underlying corporeality of the dispute. The text of the opinion piece begins with a discussion of the struggle of the Jewish people to gain control over the Wall, and the continuing Arab threat to Jewish sovereignty. "Despite [this threat] several Jewish women are of the opinion that this is the place and time to declare a sub-culture war for the desecration of the holiness of the Western Wall"

(*Yedioth Aharonoth*, November 17, 1996). For Eichler, the Women of the Wall are both unnatural (beard-growing) and dangerous to the Jewish state and Jewish sovereignty over the most sacred place on earth, two accusations that repeatedly intertwine in Israeli gendered corporeal discourse.[11]

The Women of the Wall have tried to stake a claim not only to Israel's holiest national site but also to its holiest ritual object, the Torah, which is the charter of the Jewish people and a document that grants culturally esteemed authority to those who know it well. The public presence of a group of women flagrantly disregarding traditional gender patterns and demanding their own portion of collective property certainly is enough to enrage the religious establishment. But I suspect that on a deeper level the Women of the Wall elicit such anger because they threaten a key corporeal metaphor in Jewish culture—the metonymic association between Torah and women's bodies. Traditionally, Torah scrolls like women are beautifully clothed (in crown and gown), kept hidden (housed in the ark), and undressed, opened, and deciphered by men of privilege; on Simhat Torah a wedding canopy is held over a male member of the synagogue congregation who is honored with the ritual title "groom of the Torah." By holding a Torah at the Western Wall the Women challenge the corporeal hegemony sacralized by Jewish tradition and national consensus. Women claiming the right to possess a Torah scroll are perceived to be women claiming the right to possess their own bodies, a demand that would undermine the core of patriarchal social arrangements. The Women of the Wall have consulted attorneys, raised funds, gone to court, written articles, and given speeches in which they demand that they be accorded their due rights as human beings and as Jews. But more than anything else, they have revolted against the traditional Jewish conflation of women and sacred text, both of which are subject to male control and scrutiny. By holding Torah scrolls at the Wall they have changed their ontological status from that of symbol to that of agent, a transformation that cannot but evoke fury in a culture predicated upon male ownership of the symbol system.

Another group of women who have elicited equally negative responses, and equally sexual invectives, are the Women in Black, who stand weekly silent vigils in public squares in order to denounce the Israeli occupation of Palestinian land. Their public positioning, clothed in black, can be seen as resisting not only military domination but also both the consumer culture that construes women's bodies as sites of decoration and the maternal-religious complex that assigns women's bodies to the sphere of domesticity.

Women in Black have become targets for verbal and physical violence that link gender to political conflict in dramatically corporeal ways. According to Sara Helman and Tamar Rapoport, many of the curses hurled at the Women in Black come from male taxi drivers, suggesting, it seems to me, anger at the challenge over men's (and men's vehicles) ownership of the public domain. The epithets flung at the women protesters include "fuck all of you up your ass," "you should all be fucked and then killed," "whores of Arafat," and "Arab fuckers" (1997, 690). While many of these same invectives have also been hurled at the Women of the Wall, in the context of the protests of the Women in Black against military actions they carry the additional weight of the national phobia that "our women" will be raped by enemy men (or even worse, that "our women" will prefer enemy men).[12] This sort of language explicitly ties together women's public presence to their "blatant" sexuality (the indelible mark of immutable gender) which potentially can betray the collective.

Although those who curse at the Women in Black are mostly secular while those who curse at the Women of the Wall are mostly ultra-Orthodox, both groups of cursers seem to be drawing from a shared cultural gender schema that sentences women to irredeemable corporeality. In both cases, those who disagree with a political or religious stance, pronounced by women through an action of presence in the public sphere, chose to express their disagreement by means of reference to women's physicality. At various points in the hostilities, the women's idealogical or political platforms became all but irrelevant (the Women in Black even stand silently); their very presence was sufficient to provoke anger, which, as we have seen, was directed at their bodies as much as at their ideas. While the Women of the Wall and the Women in Black may be extreme cases, it seems to me that the clarity of their conscious and purposeful physical presence has served to expose the attitudes—usually couched in the nicer language of "purity" and "modesty"—that underlie escalating efforts to supervise and control women's bodies. Reactions to the Women of the Wall and the Women in Black make explicit the intense and compelling gendered belief system that propels the skirmishes described in the rest of this chapter.

The Price of Fashion

Over the past several years, a number of local municipalities and national government offices have instituted "modest" dress codes for women workers.[13] For example, women employees of Hadera City Hall were instructed to come to work in "modest clothing" following complaints by ultra-Orthodox city councilors. The Kiryat Malachi Local Council made a similar demand on its female workers in response to complaints by men that they were being served by women in "revealing" clothing.

Ma'ariv (July 15, 1997) reported that a Knesset kiosk employee who wore a sleeveless blouse to work was told by her boss that she must come to work modestly dressed. In order to continue working that day she was forced to wear a robe over her blouse. According to reports in the press, the woman's boss yelled at her, shouting that she shamed the place and broke the rules. In response to the incident, Knesset member Shlomo Beniziri commented that he "welcomes all efforts to keep rules of modest dress so that there will be freedom of movement for religious men [*datiyim*] in the Knesset building." Beniziri added that members of his party (Shas, or Sephardi Torah Guardians) had approached the previous Knesset chair with a request to make sure that employees dress modestly in order to make "freedom of movement" (for men) possible, and that the requests were met with "good will."

In August 1996, Eliahu Suissa, an ultra-Orthodox Knesset member, was appointed Minister of Religion. Women employees at the ministry began to come to work in skirts and long-sleeved blouses, even though, according to the ministry, "they were not ordered to do so." Assuming that the ministry's claim is true (there very well may have been subtle pressure exerted on the women), this anecdote indicates how quickly women may come to take corporeal demands for granted (particularly when their jobs are at stake). Accelerating demands to cover women's bodies sometimes are met with consternation on the part of secular women, yet seldom are met with strong protest. While certain "modesty" demands are in a sense new (or at least intensified), they are consistent with a culturally recognizable metamythic language of women's corporeality already familiar to—and deemed legitimate by—many Israeli women and men. After all, the Biblical matriarch Rebecca covered her face when she met her husband Isaac.

A member of the municipal religious council of Beit She'an, Rabbi Reuven Der'i has commissioned silk "modesty capes" that "immodestly" dressed brides will be required to wear during marriage ceremonies conducted in that town. And when Meir Shabbat, owner of a bridal salon in Tiberius, submitted an advertisement to the municipal yellow pages with a picture of a bride in a wedding dress, he was told that the picture would not be printed because her shoulders were bare. According to press reports (*Ma'ariv*, May 28, 1998), the Tiberius yellow pages office confirmed that it was indeed their recent policy not to print material that could hurt "the religious public's sensitivities." We have seen how various institutions (the state, the religious establishment, and the extended family) compete for control of the bride's body; the Tiberius yellow pages story shows that merchants and the advertising industry also claim a piece of the prize.

Several supermarkets around the country have instituted dress codes for women. Typically, these dress codes mandate that women wear skirts or dresses, and blouses with sleeves. Some stores now keep a supply of skirts in the entrance so that women customers entering in slacks may cover themselves "properly" (see, for example, *Ma'ariv*, September 22, 1996). Controversy over a newly instituted modest dress policy at certain Supersol supermarkets earned extensive media attention in September 1996. The manager of the Supersol branch in question was forthright and forthcoming in his comments to the press: He wants to attract ultra-Orthodox customers to the store because they constitute a lucrative and insufficiently tapped market. Although he himself is not Orthodox, he sees the modesty policy as sound business practice. This and other similar incidents highlight the shifting relationships among the various institutions that control women's bodies; while conflict and contestation are common, in this case religion and the culture of profit-making nicely collude.

Another incident in which marketing aims and religious demands to exclude women's bodies from the public sphere teamed up occurred in August 1996, when a new post office branch was opened in the ultra-Orthodox Jerusalem neighborhood of Geula. The new branch employs only male workers to serve the public so as not "to offend the sensibilities of ultra-Orthodox customers." Postal Authority spokeswoman Sigal Galil

> defended assigning only male employees to the new branch as an appropriate marketing tactic. Prior to the branch opening, an avalanche of press releases stressed the enhanced service the authority was providing the city's ultra-Orthodox population. Galil pointed out that the Mea She'arim branch, which also serves an ultra-Orthodox population, has always had only male employees in response to customer demand. "We want them to continue being our customers." (*Jerusalem Post*, August 22, 1996)

One wonders what alternative postal service Galil is afraid ultra-Orthodox men will use.

This time the conflict settled down fairly quickly: The Israel Women's Network registered a complaint with Limor Livnat, Minister of Communications and a consistent supporter of women's rights in the Knesset, and the postal authority chairman gave an order to employ women. Still, I wish to make clear that the recurrence of incidents like this in the public discourse—whether the intentions of the various parties involved are "good" or "bad"—creates a public arena in which women's bodies are the object of incessant public debate.

Magical Mystery Tours

Over the past decade, the issue of separate seating on public buses has hit the press a number of times. In 1996, for instance, rabbis instituted separate seating on the Jerusalem to Betar route. The gendered architecture of bus separation demands, without fail, that women sit in the back and men in the front, a clear symbolic statement of gendered rank. The new policy was instituted after the road on which that particular bus travels had been improved (the tunnel roads were opened). Women previously had been urged to sit in the rear of the bus, but the old road was twisty and uncomfortable and they often felt sick in the back. With the opening of the new road, an organization by the name Va'ad Darchei Yesharim (Committee for Righteous Paths) placed *pakkachim* (inspectors) on the buses to make sure women and men sit separately. According to press reports, there had been some "incidents" between the inspectors and passengers who did not agree to the gendered seating arrangements (*Kol HaIr*, December 2, 1996). The Association for Citizen's Rights filed a complaint with the Ministry of Transportation on behalf of a number of people who live in Betar and objected to a *sadran* (usher) getting up in front of the bus and making women sit in the back. Women had complained to the Association that they found themselves treated in a "humiliating and hurtful manner." The Ministry of Transportation answered that, "Although the Ministry supervises the transport on that route, it does not know of any guidelines or instructions from the national supervisor or any other body in the Ministry of Transportation, that discriminates between women and men on that route." In other words, the Ministry of Transportation absolved itself of responsibility and allowed the coerced segregation to continue (*Ma'ariv*, December 16, 1996).

Ma'ariv (June 25, 1996) ran a story about Bus Route No. 1 in Tel Aviv, operated by the Dan Company. Passengers getting on the bus at Disengoff Street one day saw stickers ordering men to sit in front and women to sit in back. In the wake of public protest, the Dan Company explained that this particular bus is usually used in the predominantly Orthodox city of Bnei Brak, but had been sent as an extra bus on a crowded day to Tel Aviv. While from a certain perspective, "all's well that ends well" (the Dan Company explained it had made a mistake and the offending bus was taken off the Tel Aviv route), in a climate of increasing religious coercion and escalating attempts to enforce gender segregation and "modest" dress for women, this kind of incident adds to a discursive atmosphere threatening to all women. Whether or not particular passengers found the signs amusing, annoying, or infuriating, the signs served to remind women that a significant part of the population (the part that represents "tradition" and holiness) finds women's bodies polluting and intrinsically immodest.

A number of bus lines are used regularly by both ultra-Orthodox and secular Israelis. I am best acquainted with the 400 bus line that connects Jerusalem to Ramat Gan and Bnei Brak. A common scenario on the buses that originate in Bnei Brak is for ultra-Orthodox men to sit singly in the double seats in the front half of the bus. A few stops further along the line the bus becomes crowded, taking on passengers from Bar Ilan University and from a central IDF complex. Typically, women passengers—including secular women—avoid "bothering" (that is their word) the ultra-Orthodox men and move to the back of the bus rather than claim one of the front seats. Not infrequently, women stand for the entire hour or longer bus ride so as not to "bother" an ultra-Orthodox man by sitting next to him. In this scenario, standing up or sitting in the far back on an extended bus trip may literally construct ill (nauseated or exhausted) female bodies, and certainly symbolically promulgates the feeling that women's bodies are so repugnant or dangerous that their presence "bothers" pious men. Whether women internalize the sense of their own bodily menace or whether they feel embarrassed or embattled, this common bus scenario reiterates cultural themes that surely have a deleterious affect on women's overall health. In the Betar-Jerusalem bus route case, some women complained publicly about the humiliation and hurt they suffered. In general, however, women become accustomed to cultural patterns in which it is understood that women's bodies are "problematic." It is only when a new restriction on women's bodies is instituted that what has been taken for granted is revealed as hurtful. But in actuality, the sickening humiliation and hurt comprise an undercurrent—or perhaps an undertow—in which Israeli women navigate on a daily basis.

The bus battles are one (albeit particularly significant) expression of the accelerating normalization of gender segregation in Israeli society. *Yedioth Aharonoth* (July 15, 1997) reported that the management of the amusement park in the city of Safed had decided to open the park on separate days for men and women customers. The headline ran: REPRESENTATIVE OF SHAS [PARTY] ON THE CITY COUNCIL: "IT IS OUTSIDE OF THE REALM OF POSSIBILITIES THAT A YOUNG WOMAN WILL SPIN ON A MERRY-GO-ROUND AND A MAN WILL STAND UNDER HER."

Presentations in the media tend to mask men's opposition to women's presence in the public realm by dragging in the red herring of clothing style; the conflict is said to be "caused" by a woman wearing "immodest" clothing (although, as we have said, women wearing skirts to mid-calf and sleeves to the elbow have also been attacked as "immodest"). One discursive arena in which the "bare" ideological issues are made explicit is in declarations by important rabbis, some of whom are on the government payroll, that women's "immodesty" is to blame for various disasters. One such example took place in 1996 (the story was published in September 1996 in *Tsomet HaSharon*, a local newspaper). In the wake of the sudden deaths of three members of Moshav Geulim (a religiously mixed—that is, Orthodox, traditional, and secular—agricultural village in the Sharon), moshav "elders" determined that the presence of women at funerals caused the misfortunes and they ordered a ban on women attending funerals in the future.[14]

At the ever more popular *hazara bitshuva* (repentance) mass rallies[15] held throughout Israel, emotionally-stirring confessional orators who tell how they used to be a sinners but have now mended their ways are among the most popular speakers. At rallies for women, the wearing of miniskirts is typically held up as the "bad old" behavior that the repentant, modestly-dressed speaker has now abandoned. At similar rallies for men, gambling, drinking, committing crimes, and taking drugs are the "bad old" behaviors. Modest dress thus becomes construed as the mark of a righteous or repentant woman, analogous to men refraining from crime or drugs. Perhaps not surprisingly, a highlight of these women's repentance rallies is an opportunity to line up and receive a blessing and hair covering from an important rabbi or *rabbanit* (rabbi's wife).[16]

Double Voyeurism

The demands of ultra-Orthodox men regarding appropriate dress for secular women are lukewarm versions of demands made by ultra-Orthodox men on their own women, who come in for ever-increasing scrutiny of their bodies and bodily coverings. Signs around ultra-Orthodox neighborhoods proclaim, "A woman who wears immodest clothing causes the Divine Presence to depart and leads many to sin. Leading someone to sin is worse than killing him." The meaning of this discourse—aimed at women—seems twofold. Women need to be admonished to dress modestly because women are more likely to be seduced by the whims of fashion; that is, women are more morally vulnerable than men, or women's moral vulnerability is more likely to be manifested corporeally. And women's bodies—improperly covered or socialized—are dangerous to men, "causing the Divine Presence to depart" and leading "many [men] to sin."

Posters and leaflets, common in ultra-Orthodox neighborhoods, promise "free tickets to hell for women who wear wigs,[17] thin stockings, or skirts with slits." Signs also admonish women who wear noisy shoes, tight clothes, skirts that come directly below the knee, or red or other bright colors. Stockings are singled out for special scrutiny: Stockings must be of at least forty denier thickness. Women who dress "immodestly" are promised a place in hell "with [the Biblical figure] Yeraboam ben Nevat and his friends who sinned and caused Israel to sin."[18] Women's bodies thus are drawn into a national narrative through their bodies and bodily coverings. In widely distributed signs and leaflets, women who want to repent are advised to consult a *rabbanit*. The rhetoric interweaves a number of themes that are central to Israeli constructions of the female body. Women are construed as staunch consumers who allow their passion for fashion to lead them and others into sin. Women's bodies, especially when situated in the public domain, endanger the collective. And women who wish to be "healed" of their corporeal sickness are advised to submit to the authority and scrutiny of an expert (in this case a *rabbanit*, but in others a physician or a rabbi).

Ultra-Orthodox voyeurism toward women's bodies is echoed in the secular press, which seems fascinated by controversies in the religious community regarding women's hair coverings. In the secular newspaper *Ma'ariv* of September 28, 1997, we read a headline: "RABBI OVADIA [YOSEF]: A WOMAN WHO WEARS A WIG WILL BURN IN HELL." Apparently, in the course of a sermon at his synagogue, the former Sephardi chief rabbi of Israel announced that any woman who enters the synagogue wearing a wig (rather than a more "modest" hat or scarf) will be sentenced, together with her husband, to ostracism from the Jewish community. Women not only endanger men (the husband also will be punished for the woman's improper covering of her body), but also jeopardize the future of the Jewish people. According to Rabbi Yosef, "If a woman wants righteous children, she should take off the wig [and, it is understood, wear a hat or scarf]. If not, her children will be uncouth." As in the Knesset debates regarding abortion (see chapter 1), the hat versus wig dispute employs women's bodies as an ethnic battlefield. When Rabbi Ovadia Yosef decrees that wigs are not sufficiently modest and instructs the women among his followers to wear scarves instead, he is in essence declaring that Ashkenazi standards of female modesty are inadequate, and that "his" women are expected to demonstrate true piety through even greater measures of corporeal control.[19]

In *Ma'ariv*'s report, ultra-Orthodox men's surveillance of women's bodies is replicated and magnified by parallel surveillance in the secular press (secular men watch Orthodox men watch women). But it would be wrong to think that this item was newsworthy *only* because of its minor prurient appeal. In fact, Rabbi Ovadia's status as former chief rabbi, spiritual leader of the Shas political party (which holds seventeen seats in the current Knesset), and informal leader of Israel's Sephardi population imbues all of his comments with cultural authority and significance. The public nature of his remarks in synagogue serves to bring into the mainstream scrutiny of women's bodies. Rabbi Ovadia Yosef's proclamations cannot be seen as the ravings of a marginal person spouting a marginal idea; he is a highly esteemed public figure quoting rules and notions that appear in Jewish sources and that historically constitute part of the Jewish way of thinking about female bodies.

Articles in the secular press reported that ultra-Orthodox women had recently begun working as fashion models or as models in commercials, "modestly dressed and with faces obscured" (*Yedi'ot*, December 18, 1997). Apparently, while certain rabbis had given approval for ultra-Orthodox women to appear as models, this permission led to conflict in the ultra-Orthodox community; some rabbis strenuously objected to women working as models under any circumstances and others gave their approval provided that the advertisements would be published only in magazines aimed at female readers. This incident, like many others, illustrates what is actually a triple patriarchal gaze aimed at women's bodies. First, capitalist market forces elicit visual attention to women's bodies in order to sell goods and services. Second, ultra-Orthodox men debate whether it is appropriate for women to model, and if so, exactly how much and what parts of their bodies can be exposed. And finally, the secular press describes the matter in detail, complete with photos and sketches of alluring women whose faces are purposely blurred (presumably to disguise their identity) and wearing ostensibly modest but actually sexually provocative clothing (something long, but tight, for example).

Modesty among ultra-Orthodox women has become an especially controversial issue, at least in part because powerful fashion and advertising industries within a profit-driven economy have penetrated even the most religiously homogeneous social enclaves. Accelerated attention to women's dress in the ultra-Orthodox community is, among other things, a ritual response to feeling set upon by the global economy. Religious authorities obsessively monitor women's clothing because capitalism construes women's bodies as a site for spending money, whereas ultra-Orthodox Judaism construes women's bodies as a site for genetic continuity. The spate of burnings of Jerusalem bus-station shelters by ultra-Orthodox men a few years ago reflected their fury at the public display of *pictures* of women (the bus-station shelters doubled as advertising billboards) being used by the advertising industry. But the actual victims, of course, were women for whom the charred remains of the bus shelters served as a daily reminder of the threat of violence that patriarchy can, and does, hold over women's bodies.

From Voyeurs to Peeping Toms

The secular press seems especially enamored with hints of ultra-Orthodox women's sexuality (fascination with the exotic, erotic "Other" is characteristic of what Edward Said [1978] calls "Orientalism"). For instance, the secular press passed on to its readers reports originally published in ultra-Orthodox newspapers concerning Orthodox young women involved in romances with bus drivers. Since romances between *secular* young women and bus drivers are not likely to be seen as newsworthy by the secular press, the titillation that spurred these articles reflects, I believe, the chance to gaze at the exotic ultra-Orthodox female body. An article in the secular paper *Yerushalayim* (October 25, 1996) described posters and newspaper advertisements put up by the "Committee for the Purity of Our Encampment" announcing that "good, modest, and pure ultra-Orthodox girls had been seduced by bus and taxi drivers." *Yerushalayim* related the story of a daughter of an "important rabbinic family" who had been seen going out with a secular bus driver. "The couple is preparing to get engaged despite the objection of her parents." The paper quotes another rabbi whose daughter became involved with a bus driver. "Drivers pick on young ladies, attract them with all sorts of temptations, talk to them about topics that one should keep silent about . . . Women, and among them my daughter, are 'light headed' [*da'tan kala*, the well-known Talmudic phrase used to explain why women should not be taught Torah] and they are attracted by the things the drivers tell them." As a result of these incidents, the "Committee" called on people in the neighborhood to report these flirtations, and was considering putting supervisors on the buses to inform on drivers and girls who talk to each other.

Articles of this sort may seem simply to fall into the innocuous journalistic category of "human interest stories"; still, it is crucial to understand that the "human interest" is specifically focused on women's bodies. In these episodes, the ultra-Orthodox establishment exposed its interest in controlling the freedom and mobility of "their" girls' bodies (note that the arena of concern was buses and taxis, the only significant sources of mobility for ultra-Orthodox women, very few of whom drive), while the secular press exposed its prurient interest in the usually concealed bodies of ultra-Orthodox women.

The last incident I shall cite here demonstrates how easily scrutiny of women's bodies slips into out-and-out voyeurism. Secular newspapers from early December 1996 (see, for example, *Ma'ariv*, December 1, 1996) shouted the following headline: "RABBI CAUGHT A MARRIED ULTRA-ORTHODOX WOMAN ALONE WITH A BUILDING RENOVATOR." Note that the headline draws immediate attention to the man's *profession* and the woman's *religious and marital status.* The first line of the article contains a news tidbit that one would have thought interesting enough to Israeli readers to merit at least a subhead: It turns out the building contractor is an Arab! But this detail, even in Israel's highly ethnically polarized society, apparently was seen by the editors at *Ma'ariv* as substantially less interesting than the corporeal status of the woman.

The second paragraph of *Ma'ariv*'s report shares other crucial details with the (secular) reader. "Until she fell in love, the woman made a point of dressing modestly: long dresses and sleeves that hid every inch of her body, and a scarf covered her hair." Once she entered into her love affair however, "During the hours in which her husband was busy at prayer, she changed her outward appearance so much so as to be unrecognizable. A miniskirt and black stockings instead of her old clothes." The detailed attention to her clothes stands out against the absence of any mention of the man's appearance, and the extreme modesty of her regular attire ("that hid every inch of her body") invests the description of her uncovered body (miniskirt and black stockings) with a pornographic thrill.

The climax of the story came when they were caught. Apparently, her husband's brother saw her dressed in her "brazen clothing" and informed his Rabbi. "In a deserted place, at the exit from the city, the naked truth was revealed: The Rabbi peeked through the window of the [man's] truck, and discovered the pious woman and her lover engaged in intimacy that left no room for imagination." After a police chase (the police thought the Arab lover had abducted the woman) and some clarifications at the police station, the man "was allowed to return home in peace. Her return was different: Her husband left the house and announced that he would see her at the Rabbinate" (for divorce proceedings, a threat that resonates for secular women as well—all Jewish divorces in Israel are under the auspices of the all-male Orthodox rabbinate and it is not uncommon for women to fare poorly in divorce proceedings).

Central in this story is the spiraling theme of a woman's body as dangerous in its vulnerability. Even her long dresses and hair coverings couldn't keep her from romantic involvement with an Arab building contractor. In this case, the danger was twofold. First, she brought peril upon her lover: He was chased by the police and interrogated at the police station, a situation of real and recognizable danger for Arab men in Israel. Second, through clandestine extramarital relations with a man whose identity places him outside of the Jewish collectivity, she endangered the purity of future generations of that collectivity. Her identity as an ultra-Orthodox woman—that is, a woman whose body is singularly inscribed as a faithful vehicle of the patriarchal collectivity—made her treachery especially newsworthy, "proving" even to secular Israelis that women's bodies never can be trusted. Having betrayed the patriarchal trust, the body of the woman in this story became a legitimate object of public scrutiny both at the hands of the rabbis and at the hands of the secular press. If the right to uncover a woman's body represents ownership of that body, each additional garment that she removed could be construed as an additional act of collective betrayal. Note that even *Ma'ariv* did not condemn the rabbi for his candid voyeurism.

Anorexia: From Scrutiny to Sickness

In Israel, as in the United States, female beauty is equated with a level of slimness that, for most women, demands intense dietary dedication. But in

Israel, unlike in middle-class America, successful femininity is also equated with fecundity; motherhood is Israeli women's sacred national mission. For some women, reaching the desired degree of slimness reduces the likelihood of conception, forcing them to choose between two esteemed female corporeal values (that is, if they even are aware that low body weight has implications for fertility; see Pike and Striegel-Moore 1997). For most women, fecundity makes the battle for slimness even more difficult: Repeated pregnancies preclude the taut, eternally youthful female body promoted in the global media. Whichever choice a woman makes, she is likely to feel disappointment in her own body's "failure" to simultaneously present as a thin, lithe, pubescent girl *and* as a fertile, fecund mother of a family "blessed with children" (*mishpaha b'ruchat y'ladim*). In a recent study of women's health behavior in Israel, one third of women aged forty-five to seventy-five and one quarter of women aged twenty-one to forty-four reported feeling that they were fat or overweight; only 37% of the older women and 36% of the younger women felt satisfied with their bodies (cited in Ifrah 1999, 148).

Several studies have indicated that Israeli teenage girls have a particularly high incidence of eating disorders (see especially Sasson, Lewin, and Roth 1995). Most strikingly, Israeli girls have been found to rank highest of twenty-three European countries in dieting to lose weight, an "achievement" that remains steady from age eleven through age fifteen (Harel, Kaneh, and Rahav (1997).[20] By eighth grade, 10.5% of girls report dieting under the supervision of a physician, indicating that at least some of the Israeli medical establishment actively encourages the culture of dieting.[21] Significantly, while Israeli teenage boys rank high in frequency of sports activity, Israeli teenage girls rank among the lowest in Europe.

I find it particularly suggestive that Israeli psychiatrists and social workers believe there may be high rates of eating disorders among women soldiers because "the army requires women to abandon certain aspects of femininity and assume the identity of a soldier, which can threaten self-image and body image" (Mark et al. 1993, 69). Moreover, "dieting, sports, and exercise are encouraged in the army" (71). It is certainly the case that women soldiers are expected to be thin, yet thinness seems to be demanded of them for iconic reasons of neatness and attractiveness rather than because their soldiering requires it; women do not serve in combat roles and few women work at jobs that necessitate physical fitness. Thin female bodies in the IDF are congruent with the image of women soldiers as "rapeable" (weak, attractive) representatives of the state, and demonstrate—embody—the success of the military project of corporeal control. It does not surprise me to learn that anorexia is a problem in the IDF, despite the fact that girls are screened for anorexia and precluded from army service if discovered during their pre-induction physical examinations to have anorectic tendencies.

In a fascinating comparative study of ten Jewish and Arab sub-populations within Israel, it was found that kibbutz girls (more than village, city, and boarding school Jewish girls or any Arab girls) most resemble hospitalized anorectics in terms of eating attitudes and body image (Apter et al. 1994). The authors of the study point to the high role stress experienced by kibbutz women who are "expected to succeed at work (if not necessarily in a career), as a homemaker, and as an attractive, sexually desirable object" (95; see also Kaffman and Sadeh 1989). The situation of kibbutz women, it seems to me, epitomizes Robert Karasek's model of the deleterious health effects of working in jobs characterized by high responsibility and low authority. It is difficult to think of a population of women with less power than kibbutz women. From the first years of the kibbutz movement, men have dominated the leadership roles and high prestige (production) jobs, and women have worked mainly in low-status service positions (laundries, child care, kitchen, dining room). Kibbutz women cannot even exercise the forms of micro-power that go along with rationing, preparing, and serving the household's food: The kibbutz's communal menus are planned by experts, often at the level of the national kibbutz movements. As iconic "ideal" Zionists, kibbutz women carry on their shoulders the heavy burden of representing the Zionist enterprise at its agricultural apex, yet lack opportunities to contribute valued skills or talents to that enterprise. Caught between a cultural heritage of shunning bourgeois consumerism in favor of working the soil, and a social reality in which men prefer women who are attractive according to the standards of that very same shunned bourgeois consumer society, kibbutz women struggle against great odds to make corporeal statements using the few resources at their disposal. Choosing not to eat in a society in which communal eating was supposed to free women from domestic *responsibilities*, but in fact freed women only from domestic *authority*, is a corporeal statement difficult to ignore.

Orthodox and ultra-Orthodox Jewish women are similarly susceptible to the pressures placed upon women in contemporary Western societies to be thin. A recent very provocative study of ultra-Orthodox Jewish women in America suggests that the epidemic of anorexia "is particularly grave in the Orthodox world, some say because of stresses unique to the community—not least, the pressure for women to marry early, and the prevailing assumption that thin women get the best catches" (Haas 1999, 28). In the ultra-Orthodox world of matchmaking, a woman's physical appearance (slim, neat, attractive, and modest) is capital that can be traded on the marriage market for men of highest value: Torah scholars.

Yet it seems to me that anorexia among Orthodox Jewish women has to do with some additional factors that may further exacerbate the modern secular cult of female thinness. In previous chapters I have argued that women's bodies tend to function as cultural symbols; their bodies are "read" for inscribed messages. The emaciated body of the anorectic certainly carries some very visible cultural messages. In secular Western society those messages may include the demise of social esteem for traditional avenues of female success and self-worth (maternity, housework); the anorectic body may look childlike or it may look genderless, but it certainly does not look fecund and maturely feminine. In the context of Orthodox Jewish culture, the anorectic body can be read as the perfect modest woman's body, a body that has successfully conquered the "messiness" of femininity through erasure of feminine curves and the cessation of menstruation. The anorectic girl is unquestionably pure: asexual and amenstrual.

As we have seen throughout this chapter, the ultimate measure of female corporeal value in the Orthodox Jewish world is modesty. The "problem" is that modesty is an elusive, subjective, and changeable state, shifting throughout the life cycles of individuals and throughout the generations in accordance with and in reaction to "outside" fashions and modesty standards (we saw this earlier in the arguments regarding wigs versus scarves). Demands for modesty tend to elicit extensive corporeal scrutiny and control, both on the part of authorities (parents, teachers, rabbis) and on the part of girls and women themselves. Similarly, issues of scrutiny and control stand out in the psychological literature on anorexia (Gordon 1990, 123–124): The anorectic girl has perfectly interiorized the intense cultural gaze directed at women's bodies, at the same time that she has reached the ultimate heights of corporeal control. What I believe has taken place in Orthodox and ultra-Orthodox communities is the convergence of traditional Jewish techniques for managing female corporeality, with a modern "syndrome" that has proven capable of crossing subcultural borders.

For Orthodox Jews, modesty is far more than a matter of clothing. Modesty, especially in women, has to do with corporeal deportment in every sense. (Thus, for example, some ultra-Orthodox rabbis forbid women to wear red clothes because red's brightness is "immodest.") As we have seen in this chapter, modesty for traditional Jewish women is often conceptualized in terms of presence: Regardless of what clothes are worn, women's visible or audible presence (especially, but not only, in the public sphere) tends to be defined as intrinsically immodest. Women's presence does not even need to be in the flesh; *pictures* of women were burned in the bus shelter incidents described earlier. Pushing this point a bit further, it seems to me that the anorectic body is the least "present" that a female body can be: Anorectic women have trained their bodies to take up very little space. Protracted self-starvation erases markers of female corporeality—

an attractive feat in a misogynistic world. But carried to its extreme it can do even better than that; self-starvation can make women altogether and irreversibly invisible—the ultimate in female modesty.

An additional point of convergence takes place between traditional Jewish rituals of controlling food (prohibiting certain foodstuffs, separating dairy from meat products and the utensils used to cook them, removing a portion of bread dough as a symbol of sacrifice, and so on) and anorectic rituals of food control (cutting food up into certain size pieces, putting large quantities of mustard or vinegar on food, prohibiting certain foods; see O'Halloran 1993, 137–138; Crisp 1995, 80; Bruch 1978, 8–9). Significantly, whereas strict adherence to Jewish food rituals prompts women to seek the expert advice and accept the expert control of rabbis, strict adherence to anorectic food rituals prompts women to seek the expert advice and accept the expert control of doctors and psychologists. In the case of anorectic women, the final irony is that the prescribed treatment for a disorder characterized by "neurotic" self-scrutiny (for thinness) consists of unrelenting, highly intrusive, yet allegedly "legitimate" scrutiny by members of the medical institution (checking that the "patient" has eaten, gained weight, not induced vomiting, and so on). The cure, it seems to me, bears an uncanny resemblance to the disorder, hinting that both are products of the same very deeply embedded gender conceptualizations.

Anorexia among ultra-Orthodox women, kibbutz women, and women soldiers is of particular interest because of the iconic value of these women as representatives of Judaism, Zionism, and the state. Yet I am convinced that the cultural project of incessant scrutiny of *all* women's bodies has serious consequences for Israeli women across the subcultural divides. Many of us have had the experience of staring at our own feet or fingers until they no longer feel as if they are "us" but rather seem to be foreign, disembodied objects. Incessant scrutiny transforms the scrutinized body into an object to be gazed at rather than a subject with the power to gaze—a perception that comes to be shared by the scrutinizer and the scrutinized alike. This process reaches fruition in anorectic behavior and its medicalized treatment, but lies beneath the surface of the corporeal experiences of all Israeli women.

Conclusion

Resisting Bodies

So Chana says: "God gives death and life, draws down to Sheol and raises up. God impoverishes and makes wealthy, humbles and also exalts." What is meant by "also [*'af*] exalts?" By the fury [*'af*] which he brings upon one, he exalts another. A matron asked Rabbi Shimon ben Halafta: "How many days did it take God to make the world?" He responded: "Six days" . . . She said to him, "And from then until now, what has He been doing?" He responded: "He sits and makes hierarchies [*sulamot*]—exalting one and humbling another."

—BAMIDBAR RABBA, Seder Mattot, 8[1]

The preceding chapters have exposed some of the multiple layers of institutional authority that shape Israeli women's corporeal experiences, depriving them of authority while heaping responsibility on their shoulders and wombs. We have seen how medical, religious, military, economic, and state institutions engage in multifarious projects of collusion and competition to control women's bodies. In Israeli culture women's bodies are constructed as symbolic capital or resources to be fought over, and battlegrounds to be fought on. Yet despite the compelling collaboration of a variety of powerful institutions, women do sometimes transform themselves from symbol to agent, and resist popular constructions.

Throughout this book examples of women's resistance have been noted: demonstrations by Ministry of Education employees, refusal to ride in the back of a bus that travels on twisted roads, scathing comments by women Knesset members, interviews with the press in which women identify ultra-Orthodox religious coercion as their "real enemy" and Arabs as their allies, insistence upon serving in traditional male roles in the IDF, and complaints filed against sexually abusive men, including military officers. These are all significant acts of resistance, demonstrating both conceptual critique of widely accepted popular discourses and instrumental actions aimed at changing specific oppressive situations.

When we read through such a stunning list of women's acts of resistance, it may be difficult to understand why gender hierarchy remains such a potently oppressive force in Israeli culture. The dilemmas that confront feminist scholars writing about women's resistance have been summed up well by Kathy Davis and Sue Fisher:

> On the one hand, if we focus on asymmetrical social structures, we tend to lose sight of how women produce and reproduce but also resist and undermine these structures. We then run the risk of treating women as if they are passive victims of repressive systems. On the other hand, if we focus on women's agency, we often fail to locate this agency within a social and/or political context. Here if women resist but are not successful, we run the risk of blaming the victim—of attributing responsibility to women for conditions over which they often have little control. (1993, 4)

Taking a middle ground, in the discussion that follows I have tried to situate women's resistance as one factor in the shifting dialectical relationships among the various institutions that comprise Israeli society.

Institutional Ping-Pong

When Israeli women resist the practices of one powerful gendering institution, they frequently find themselves smack in the gendered arms of another equally powerful institution. For example, we have seen throughout this book that some Israeli women respond to oppression by becoming ill. Women's somatic symptoms can be considered a form of resistance to patriarchal demands: Somatization can expose the harmful reality of living with oppression (that is certainly one of the effects of the current epidemic of anorexia) and illness sometimes gives women time out from the responsibilities and stress that may be making them sick. Karen Pliskin illustrates this scenario among Iranian women in Israel:

> For some women . . . the label of rheumatism allows them to take time off washing clothes and dishes, leaving the responsibility to others, or leaving the work undone. Women are particularly prone to pains in their arms, and it is customary to complain about the pains in a high-pitched voice and rub the afflicted arm with the one that feels normal, and to attribute the pains to years of housework for their families, or to an unknown agent. (1987, 148)

Moreover, according to Pliskin, women are eager to go to doctors to get a diagnosis of rheumatism, which legitimates both their pain and their rest from housework.

This strategy, it seems to me, offers women a certain respite from the demands of work and family, but at the high price of collusion with negative and patriarchal conceptualizations of female corporeality (not to mention negative conceptualizations of North African and Asian Jews). Women's "time out" comes at the expense of pain, suffering, and publicly acceding to cultural beliefs regarding women's inherent sickness and weakness. And above all, it sends women into the clinics and waiting rooms of the gendered and gendering medical establishment, thus reinforcing women's dependence upon medical experts.

The depth and breadth of the patriarchal grasp means that women's resistance, despite the best of intentions, often acknowledges or actually enhances the legitimacy of the very institutions that oppress women. Even the women enacting one of the most dramatic examples of resistance we have seen—the Women of the Wall who battle for the right to hold a Torah at the Western Wall—accept and indeed glorify the symbolic and political power of a document that sanctifies and naturalizes gender difference and male dominance ("Your desire shall be to your husband and he will rule over you" [*Genesis* 3:16]). Similarly, it seems to me that the struggle of women to serve in combat units should be viewed with some ambivalence. It is certainly true that the exclusion of women from roles of authority and prestige in the IDF perpetuates negative images of women in general and prevents women from attaining positions of authority in the political system in particular. However, it is also true that including women in combat blurs the patriarchal nature of the military enterprise and the violent nature of the patriarchal enterprise. Women volunteering for combat (and women insisting that other women be conscripted into combat positions) may lead to particularly hurtful forms of collusion with the patriarchal-military complex—thus camouflaging the complex's historical program of gendered violence and domination.

The might of patriarchy is that it embeds its conceptualizations in the very bodies of the men and women whose lives it governs. The power that fuels gender hierarchies is "continuous, subtle, and productive . . . It is a 'capillary' circulating through the social body and exerting its authority through self-surveillance and everyday, disciplinary micropractices—practices [even] more fundamental than beliefs (ideology). These practices insinuate themselves within gestures, habits, bodies, and desires" (Davis and Fisher 1993, 8). Patriarchy indeed makes women sick, but resisting patriarchy can look or feel as if it tears apart the bodies that we have become accustomed to. Resistance can be enormously liberating, and it can be excruciatingly painful.

Women's acts of corporeal resistance sometimes look to observers as if they are harmful to the resister herself. Thus women may resist conceptualizations that depict the female body as eternally harboring invisible, pernicious cancer cells (in all of its most female organs, of course) by "forgetting" to go for mammograms or to practice breast self-examination. Young women may resist double standards for male and female sexuality by engaging in "promiscuous" sexual activity. Cross-culturally women (and other subordinate groups) use the platforms available to them to make public or private statements of resistance. For women, the choice of platforms often is small; there are few resources or arenas that they control, and their own bodies may well be the only valued property that they are free to manipulate. Thus some women may resist the cultural demand that women be slim and attractive by choosing eating behaviors leading to corpulence or, alternatively, eating behaviors labeled anorexia. I find it significant that psychologists see issues of control standing at the center of anorectic food behaviors. Gordon, for instance, writes that, "They [anorectics] are driven to the behavior almost wholly from a sense of intolerable dependence and enmeshment . . . The fierce struggle for self-control and a sense of power in anorexia is actually rooted in a profound sense of powerlessness" (1990, 124–125). Choosing not to eat, as "unhealthy" as that may be, is an expression of control in situations in which few other choices are available.

Before entering into a more detailed exploration of gendered resistance in Israeli society, I wish to clarify that from my point of view as an anthropologist, these acts of resistance are as legitimate as any others. Who am I to say whether in the long run it is better for women to diet than to eat what they wish, to annually offer up their breasts to sophisticated x-ray probes or to avoid the extra dose of radiation, to seek sexual adventure or to guard their "purity"? My goal here is not to judge the value of various endeavors to resist gender hierarchy; it is simply to draw attention to the complexities involved in deconstructing a patriarchal system that involves such a large variety of powerful, persuasive, and tenacious institutions.

Reflecting back on the institutional constructions explored in previous chapters, we turn now to a number of situations that show how difficult it can be for women to break out of the patriarchal maze with its power to both possess and prepossess (Daly 1978).

Abortion

Israeli women resist the state's intrusive requirements for obtaining legal abortions. First and foremost, many women (the exact numbers are unknown, but believed to be high) circumvent the government-mandated committees that approve or deny abortions by paying privately for what is known as a "gray" abortion—an abortion that is neither legal nor actively prosecuted by the police or courts. Gray abortions are widely available and usually carried out safely and hygienically by licensed physicians. But the price is high; gray abortions have turned into a comfortable money-making proposition for many Israeli physicians. The cost, of course, is borne by women. In a typical Israeli pattern, women do have access to a certain degree of autonomy, women do manage to free themselves from the jurisdiction of state institutions, but in order to do so they embrace—at a significant financial cost—profit-making medicine in a country that prides itself on its low-cost, accessible, national health services.

Other women resist the abortion law by deceiving the abortion committees. With the repeal in 1979 of the clause allowing abortions on socioeconomic grounds, the number of approved abortions did *not* decrease, suggesting that women began using other clauses in the law to obtain abortions. A government publication presents statistics on women who approached the pregnancy termination committees from 1988 through 1994 (*Selected Characteristics* 1996). As the years went on, fewer women were turned down; women seem to be getting savvier at knowing what to tell the committees.

Yet this form of resistance also has a cost. The remaining clauses in the abortion law limit legal abortions to women who are defined as sick physically, psychologically, or socially (a victim of "forbidden sexual relations"). There is no clause that allows a healthy women who wishes to terminate a pregnancy to do so. Yishai (1997, 221) reports that in 1979, 39.7% of approvals in abortion committees were granted on the basis of the socioeconomic clause; following its repeal, the number of those granted permission on health grounds increased five-fold (from 1,299 to 5,796). Thus even women who resist the abortion law through the use of creative discursive maneuvers (often learned through an informal women's underground), become complicit in the cultural construction of women's reproductive lives as inherently unhealthy.

Multiple Models of Childbirth

As we saw in chapter 2, a fair number of Israeli women resist the medicalized approach to childbirth legislated by the Knesset and thrust on women by doctors and hospitals. Yet the most prevalent form of resistance is the embrace of blessings and amulets distributed by holy men and rabbis who subscribe to gender systems that are equally if not more hierarchical and authoritarian than the medical establishment.

Most of the Jerusalem women I interviewed made use of more than one model of childbirth. The selection of a mixture of formal Jewish rituals, folk religious rituals, modern medical rituals, and natural childbirth breathing rituals means that women are involved with multiple sorts or sources of authority—doctors, midwives, childbirth education teachers, and rabbis. On the one hand, by turning to multiple sources of authority the women seem to suggest that they do not have total faith in, or allegiance, to any one particular source. Calling up a rabbi to consult with him when a doctor orders a cesarian section can be seen as an empowering expression of resistance to the authority of the dominant medical institution. On the other hand, it can be argued that phone calls of that sort are disempowering expressions of the hold of multiple sources of authority—of competing sources of control engaged in spiraling competition for power over women's bodies.

Writing about women and infertility in contemporary China, Lisa Handwerker observed that,

> If a diagnosis did not conform to a woman's explanatory model, she would often seek out another health practitioner until she found one whose beliefs coincided with her own. Also, most peasant women admitted to seeking out services and engaging in practices that are considered "feudalistic" or superstitious by the CCP such as practicing *feng shui*, praying to Kuan Yin, the Goddess of Mercy, and/or eating dyed red eggs at a wedding to increase fertility. Such practices represent a challenge to the party-state that equates science with truth. (1998, 195)

Handwerker argues that infertile women's use of a number of systems may be viewed as counterhegemonic, reflecting competing moralities that persist between individuals and the state.

While I certainly agree with Handwerker that folk religious practices undermine the monolithic power of the state, it is not at all clear to me that reverting to "feudalistic" mystifying practices constitutes feminist resistance. Not only do I (like many other feminist scholars) see significant lines of continuity between medieval, modern, and postmodern forms of patriarchy, but in the Israeli case in particular the level of cooperation between the male-dominated medical and religious establishments is so high that they often enhance rather than detract from one another's power. Trained in subordination to one institution, women may easily accept a subordinate role in another.

The Wig Revolution

Secular Israeli women who reject the commodification of female sexuality sold by the media and fashion industry sometimes choose to run into the comforting arms of Orthodox rules of female modesty and purity. Ironically, the reverse is also true: Orthodox women who evade the rabbis' regulation of women's clothing tend to run right into the equally greedy arms of the fashion industry.

One of the more persistent forms of corporeal resistance to dominant constructions of women's bodies is carried out by Orthodox and ultra-Orthodox women who continually push the limits of "modest" dress codes. Among young Orthodox women in the 1990s, for example, it has been fashionable to wear modestly long skirts, but with slits up the back. This sort of limit-pushing constitutes an ongoing undercurrent of contestation between women and rabbis, never erupting into organized defiance on the part of women, yet stubbornly present as a reminder of the possibility of female corporeal challenge to the patriarchal status quo.

Tracing changes over the years in women's clothing and hair covering customs in her native ultra-Orthodox Bnei Brak community, Sheri Makover (*Ma'ariv*, November 19, 1997) explains that when she was a young girl, Bnei Brak women wore modest and plain clothes and covered their hair with scarves or blatantly artificial-looking wigs. Now, however, the women dress in lovely purchases from boutiques and wig studios. The transformation in women's clothing is something that the rabbis have not been able to thwart. Magazines for Orthodox women are replete with attractive fashion advertisements (in which the clothes are shown on dummies or hangers instead of models), ultra-Orthodox women attend fashion shows, and a good suit to wear on the Sabbath can easily cost 1,500 to 2,000 shekels ($350 to $500), dresses for weddings and other occasions as much as 6,000 shekels ($1,500, easily one and a half month's salary for an ultra-Orthodox woman).

Makover especially notes what she calls the "wig revolution." Whereas the rabbis have not objected very vocally to the fashion revolution (they don't like it but they have not taken strong steps to prohibit it), they have objected repeatedly and vociferously to wigs (see chapter 5). A number of wig salons have been the target of arson attacks, and posters in ultra-Orthodox neighborhoods warn women not to patronize the salons. Yet Makover was told by the owner of a wig salon that, "The [ultra-Orthodox] women and also their husbands want women who look natural and young." As a result, since Rabbi Ovadia Yosef ruled that wigs are improper, large numbers of Asian and North African ultra-Orthodox women "have turned into consumers of fashionable hats." The women buy hats for different seasons and different occasions, and styles change quite often. An inexpensive hat for everyday use costs 60 to 80 shekels ($15 to $20), nice hats for weddings and holiday celebrations cost 200 to 400 shekels ($50 to $100).

What Makover in fact describes are ongoing acts of corporeal resistance on the part of ultra-Orthodox women. They are told to wear modest clothes, so they wear beautiful, fashionable, expensive modest clothes. They are told to cover their hair, so they wear glamorous, luxurious wigs.

They are told that wigs are insufficient, so they buy expensive, fashionable hats. Yet their resistance to the corporeal constructions of the religious establishment has sent them straight into the corporeal constructions of the capitalist marketplace, and especially the multibillion-dollar fashion industry. In resisting one problematic construction, women have embraced another. Looking fashionable, glamorous, and above all "young," takes a toll on women's health and psyches no less than looking "modest" does.

Mikveh

The eagerness with which many Orthodox, traditional, and secular women in Israel observe the rituals of niddah and mikveh and embrace the gendered corporeal conceptualizations that are expressed by those rituals suggests that other available conceptualizations of the female body may be even less attractive to them. In the current mikveh literature, the "pure" woman and her happy and viable family are contrasted to the commodified, perpetually sexually exploited, emotionally and economically vulnerable, modern Western woman. By opting for menstrual purity and sexual restraint, some women set out to resist the Western profit-making/fashion/pornographic construction of female corporeality.

Most of the Beer Sheva women in Inbal Cicurel's study said they themselves had chosen to observe niddah and mikveh, a smaller group said it was a joint decision of husband and wife, and only a scant few said the husband requested it. In my own work I have heard many woman say that their husbands actively oppose their keeping the laws of niddah and resent the two-week sexual separation. (Ashkenazi mikveh attendants will often try to "strengthen" Asian and North African women in their resolve to wait the full two weeks before resuming sexual activity despite pressure from their husbands—another example of competition over women's bodies). Some women experience observing the laws of menstrual (im)purity as a means of maintaining some sense of control over their own sexuality and a means of resisting cultural expectations that husbands will have unlimited sexual access to their wives. Rahel Wasserfall has shown that some women capitalize on mikveh observance to negotiate emotional or economic advantages within the marital relationship (1990). For many women, the mikveh building serves as a female enclave in which they are, for a time, free of the demands of husbands, bosses, small children, and elderly parents.

Commitment to observing the laws of niddah and mikveh indeed loosens the hold that certain powerful institutions—the heterosexual family and the Western consumer economy—have on women. But in the usual Israeli pattern, it does so by strengthening the hold of another institution, the religious establishment. The niddah and mikveh discourse of the religious establishment seems to offer women dignified alternatives to ceaseless sexual availability and the Western commodification of sexuality. Yet the corporeal price is very high. By submitting to the authority of the religious establishment, women can become (temporarily) pure, but that submission entails acknowledging that without the purifying powers of the religious establishment, women in their natural state embody pollution, danger, and sickness.[2]

Gatekeepers

In the case of the niddah and mikveh ritual complex, women's submission is mediated through other women, who serve as gatekeepers and institutional representatives. Nira Yuval-Davis notes:

> [W]hen we consider the political implications of the ways women are constructed as biological reproducers of "the nation"... [V]ery often it is [other] women, especially older women, who are given the roles of the cultural reproducers of "the nation" [and] are empowered to rule on what is "appropriate" behavior and appearance and what is not, and to exert control over other women who might be constructed as "deviants." (1997, 37)

Mary Daly similarly draws attention to the role of women ritual officiants in a whole range of cultural practices (such as footbinding and infibulation) in which women's bodies are manipulated, purified, or otherwise improved. The irony is that in many cases these kinds of positions are the only leadership positions available to women who are ambitious, assertive, outgoing, talented, zealous, determined, or strong-natured. It is not unusual for women to choose these positions out of an earnest desire to "make things better" and to serve other women. Yet once in these positions, women—even the stoutest of heart—tend to become part of the well-oiled machine of patriarchy. Resistance from within is tricky indeed.

There are important parallels between the mikveh attendant (and the mother-in-law) in the prenuptial mikveh ritual, midwives who attend births, social workers on abortion committees, and even Women's Army Corps officers. All of these women are front-line representatives of patriarchal institutions in which they themselves hold little or no power. These women serve as gatekeepers to institutions upon whose services Israeli women are dependent, and their presence serves to mask the gendered hierarchy of the institutions and deflect women's anger away from the elite men who are truly in charge. Despite sporadic episodes of camaraderie between women gatekeepers and their women clients, the relationship is one that functions to turn women against women, and obscures the true sources of oppressive and sickening policies, regulations, ideologies, attitudes, and practices.

The social worker on abortion committees spends far more time questioning women who request abortions than the two doctors do and she is the committee member who tends to be perceived as helpful or unhelpful, overly inquisitive or not, when in fact she is outnumbered two to one on the abortion committee, did not design either the law or its implementation mechanism, and holds little actual power. Midwives tend to be perceived as having the power to grant or withhold pain-killing medication and are praised or blamed for how the birth turns out, although it is doctors, not midwives, who set hospital policy in matters concerning childbirth.[3] Women in the IDF officially belong to the Women's Army Corps and Women's Army Corps officers have exclusive judiciary authority over women; only they can judge women accused of any military offense, although most complaints come from the males under whom the women are working (see Yuval-Davis 1985, 661). Women's Army Corps officers can easily bear the brunt of the anger of women soldiers reprimanded or punished for a military offense, despite the fact that the Women's Army Corps has negligible institutional power within the IDF.

Thus, in the case of compulsory mikveh immersion of Israeli brides, the male rabbis who make and adjudicate the laws, the male members of the Knesset who voted to give religious authorities control of weddings, and the husband and his father who are the true members of the lineage into which the bride is marrying are absent from the bride's mikveh encounter. They leave it up to their womenfolk—to the mother-in-law and the mikveh attendant—to carry out the actual physical procedures upon the bride's body. Mary Daly suggests that the use of women as "scapegoats" and "token torturers" functions to "mask the male-centeredness of the ritualized atrocity and turn women against each other" (1978, 132). On a deeper level, by turning women against one another, women are turned against themselves.

The resentment of the secular bride is likely to be directed at the mikveh attendant rather than at the government or the *halacha* (Jewish law) that has set up the mikveh attendant as an agent or scapegoat. This may explain why it has become commonplace in Israel for secular brides to trick or avoid the mikveh attendant,[4] yet there has been no organized resistance to the entire coercive ritual complex. The presence of women as gatekeepers (and bear in mind that the women gatekeepers, generally underpaid for their work, are probably struggling to resist their own economic disempowerment) tends to foil possibilities for meaningful resistance.

Maternal Politics

Up to now we have looked primarily at private acts of resistance carried out by individual women struggling to get by, survive, carve out a bit of space for themselves, and improve their own lives and the lives of those with whom they closely live. Turning to women engaged in more communal, politicized, and public forms of resistance, we shall see even more clearly the interlocking power of images, structures, and paradigms propagated by the various institutions that frame Israeli women's experiences.

Living in a militarized society has numerous ill effects upon women's freedom, safety, sense of self, and health. Rape and the threat of rape, idealization of the male combatant, legitimization of male political leadership because only men "really" understand the security situation, and mothers' worry and grief over soldier-sons are but some of the deleterious aspects of militarization for women. For all of these reasons, I see resistance to the military project as a crucially important form of feminist resistance, and one in which Israeli women have increasingly chosen to engage.

The symbolic valence of the maternal body is so deeply accepted in Israeli culture that even when women wish to exercise political agency in the public realm they are likely to call on the iconic maternal body (instead of, or in addition to, other kinds of resources) to authenticate their claim to influencing the national agenda. During the past two decades, motherhood has become a brand of identity politics both for women on the political left and women on the political right (see El-Or and Aran 1995 on settler women). The Four Mothers group, for example, has called for Israeli withdrawal from Lebanon, invoking not their political acumen but rather their role as compassionate mothers, symbolic of mothers throughout Israel who suffer on behalf of their sons. A group called Women and Mothers for Peace, active in 1996–1997, explained that they were not allied with any other organization because they had a unique prerogative as women whose sons are serving, or will serve in the IDF in the future (*Jerusalem Post*, February 21, 1997).

Women for the Sanctity of Life is a recently formed group of Orthodox women whose first political act was a demonstration, held on the afternoon before Yom Kippur of 1997, in favor of the peace process and against remaining in Lebanon. *HaAretz* ran an interview with one of the organizers, Suny Bing, a Jerusalem social worker and the mother of four sons. In her comments Bing drew political legitimacy, her very right to speak, from her identity as the mother of four sons, two currently serving in the IDF. Contrasting her own concern for children with an unnamed "influential rabbi's" concern for the Biblical patriarchs buried in Hebron, she presented herself as a mother par excellence: She herself was willing to leave her own parents in Switzerland in order to raise her children in Israel, and she is willing to leave the tombs in Hebron in order to save Israeli sons. For Bing, maternity and maternal discourse open the door to challenging not only military and government policy, but also rabbinic authority. Like other women's organizations, Women for the Sanctity of Life stress that their point of departure is not a political agenda but rather a moral and human one. Tsviya Greenfield, one of the group's leaders, declared that, "It is because we are wives and mothers that we can say these terrible things: We are constantly treading in pools of blood." Drawing on potent mythic images of motherhood, Greenfield explained that the sanctification of land that has become so central to Orthodox groups in Israel today is "completely alien to authentic traditional Judaism . . . Rachel, Our Mother, wept over her sons, not the land" (*HaAretz*, October 15, 1997).

When women use the maternal body to legitimate their special brand of political involvement, they are, it seems to me, engaged in a process of claiming the right to capitalize on the symbol "mother," rather than challenging accepted cultural understandings of "motherhood" as a symbolic resource. While the issues are somewhat different when women use their own bodies as cultural symbols than when patriarchal society writ large uses women's bodies as cultural symbols, in both cases women's bodies are construed in terms of iconic value rather than in terms of agency—a construction that does not strike me as particularly health enhancing. Although the maternal discourse does depict women's bodies as symbolizing a special brand of nobility and purity, purity is not the same as power or agency, and in fact the maternal body is typically cast by women protesters as weak and sick. Maternal nobility does not, in the real world, bestow authority or strength.

Somatic symptoms experienced by mothers of soldiers have become a central part of women's discourse of resistance to militarization. Yvonne Deutsch quotes women peace activists who describe the corporeal dimensions of their conflicted and helpless feelings about their sons' service in the occupied territories:

> About a year before her eldest son was to be drafted into the army [during the Lebanon war], Miriam felt engulfed by anxiety and began to wake up in the middle of the night with nightmares. "I went to sleep as I normally do, but I woke up at 3:30 in the morning, in a cold sweat, my heart pounding fiercely. I will never forget it . . . During the day I would function; however, every night at between 3:30 and 4:00 A.M. I would wake up with those same symptoms of cold sweat, fast heartbeats and most distressing thoughts." (1994, 99–100)

While I think it is crucial for women to publicly declare that militarization makes them sick, framing resistance in terms of corporeal weakness seems to me, once again, to be a case of the frying pan and the fire. Militarization makes women sick, but resisting militarization on a platform of illness deflates and undermines women's claim to political authority by embracing a gender identity of weakness and illness, not to mention by sending women to the couches of psychologists and the examining tables of physicians.

Perhaps not surprisingly, public reaction to maternal identity politics has not been entirely supportive. Nurit Gilat examined one of the earliest maternal antiwar organizations, Parents Against Silence, which formally existed from May 1983 to July 1985 and at its peak reached about six hundred members.[5] Although Parents Against Silence resolutely insisted that their membership included both men and women, and they were adamant that their organization's name was *Parents* Against Silence, the press quickly dubbed the group *Mothers* Against Silence—a name that stuck. Many of the group's leaders indeed were women, but more than that I suspect that their reliance upon a conciliatory maternal discourse (for example, "Our criticism is not against the IDF but against those who send our sons to Lebanon" [*Al Ha-Mishmar*, May 20, 1983; cited in Gilat 1987, 24]), rather than upon open political resistance, made it easy for the press to tag them as a "mothers" group. It was then relatively simple for the media to write them off as mothers worried about their own sons serving in Lebanon rather than concerned about issues of State (26–27).

Resisting militarization through embracing a discourse of maternity has not been a successful strategy. Maternity is not construed as giving women metapersonal political acumen, but rather as blinding them to the needs of the collective because of their (understandable) devotion to their own children. One Knesset member declared in regard to Parents Against Silence that, "We are not speaking here of women, but of mothers whose feelings are understandable, but government policy cannot be decided by them" (*HaAretz*, January 1, 1984). Other statements were less moderate, contrasting mothers (irrational) to the IDF (expert and objective). An editorial in *Hadashot* (April 21, 1985) proclaimed:

> The Mothers [*sic*] Against Silence have a part in every casualty, and to the ladies of Mothers Against Silence it is our wish to say: You have a part in every casualty who fell in the last month and a half. You have a part in every road accident that took place on the road in Lebanon—that is the opinion of reserve duty officers who finished their military service the day before yesterday.

Once again, when officers and mothers were placed on the scale of public opinion, the words of mothers proved to carry little cultural weight.

In Israeli public discourse, women's motherhood and men's soldiering are said to be equal national missions. While this kind of sentiment may sound good in speeches in the Knesset, it simply is not true: Strength and weakness, health and illness, are not equal social identities. It is suggestive that until 1994 women's paid maternity leave gave them only three quarters of their actual salaries, while men on reserve duty receive 100% of their salaries. The "motherhood and soldiering" discourse, in fact, has more to do with oppositions than with equivalencies. If the male soldier-body is courageous, healthy, and strong, the mother is literally worried sick. If soldiers give their bodies for the collective, mothers are concerned with their own sons. Motherhood does not translate into real political power for women; generals, not mothers, are elected prime minister.

Equal Rights Law

The problem of being squeezed between a rock and a hard place came to the fore a few months ago in the wake of Knesset approval of an amendment expanding the 1951 Equal Rights Law. In press reports at the time, optimism engendered by the law was largely eclipsed by critical discussions of the process through which Yael Dayan, the Chair of the Knesset Committee on the Status of Women, managed to get it passed by the Knesset. Apparently, in order to gain the support (or, more precisely, to defuse the opposition) of the ultra-Orthodox Shas party, Dayan surrendered her place on the Knesset Security and Foreign Affairs Committee (probably the most important and influential Knesset Committee, and one to which women have had very little access) to (male) Shas representative Yair Peretz. In addition, Dayan agreed to remove from the bill a section that guaranteed women's freedom regarding abortion and a section that Shas claimed would lead to state recognition of marriages prohibited by Orthodox Jewish law.

Critics of Dayan's deal with the Shas party immediately argued that the new amendment will not substantively improve upon the 1951 law: Both are proclamations of general principles rather than blueprints for building a just society; the previous law was not enforced thus there is no reason to think that this one will be either; and the specific omissions from the new law (marriage and abortion) actually reify and fortify Israel's two-tier gender system (in which women are, officially, equal to men in civil matters but unequal in matters assigned to the sphere of authority of the Orthodox establishment).

The new law may, of course, turn out to be an effective piece of legislation, and I, like other Israeli women, certainly hope that it does. Yet, as of May 2000, public conversations regarding the process of passing the law have replayed patterns of collusion and competition over the right to define women's bodies, reiterated discourses of trade-offs between women and the state, and reinscribed traditional scripts of gender equality faltering at the threshold of corporeal freedom for women. Consistent with the Israeli pattern of according women symbolic honor but little real authority, it may well be that Dayan exchanged a position of actual power on the Knesset Security and Foreign Affairs Committee for a gesture of equality stripped of the very sections that could have unraveled the cultural code that restricts women's coproreal freedom.

Breaking the Cycle

The gender conceptualizations that generate Israeli women's ill health are disguised by thick symbolic trappings, naturalized through references to supposedly immutable biological "facts," and vigorously reinforced through the collaboration of all major social institutions. If what makes women sick is exclusion from positions of authority, idealization of the normative citizen-fighter-farmer as a healthy male, and cultural images of women's bodies as rape-able, impure, and prone to illness, it should be clear that opening another clinic or "getting" more women to come for mammograms will not solve the problem. Israeli women's poor health is rooted in the institutionalization of gender patterns that consistently and programmatically deny women access to power, while at the same time holding them responsible for the continuity and the purity of the collective. These patterns have been shaped by Israel's location in the highly militarized Middle East, the devastating legacy of the Holocaust, several thousand years of Jewish myth, ritual, and history, Israel's unavoidable (and often quite desirable) membership in the worldwide consumer economy, and the dramatic scientific discoveries of the twentieth century that have made the medicalization of women's bodies such a tempting cultural enterprise.

Although I do not think that effective resistance is impossible, I do think that it demands committed metafeminist analysis that focuses on multiple key links in the patriarchal chain, while all the time vigilantly checking and rechecking how the loosening of one link ricochets throughout the whole system. Ethnicity, age, and class confound one-dimensional gender analysis, at the same time that political, family, religious, military, and medical institutions merge and diverge in complex and highly charged ways.

While the picture that I have drawn in this book is not an optimistic one, I do think that there are certain arenas in which feminist activism is likely to foment and foster change. Israeli women already have access to some very important social resources which have been and certainly can continue to be drawn upon as part of an effective feminist program. The multiple ideological systems that I have traced throughout this book indeed offer one another "back up"—creating a patriarchal bulwark that is difficult to dismantle. Yet the existence of multiple systems also has the potential to liberate thought, to open conceptual cracks, to create dissonance, and to show up a patriarchal ideology or institution for the cultural creation it is rather than for the natural inevitability it claims to be.

Israeli women boast a strong tradition of women's organizations and an eagerness to organize both at the national level (for example, Na'amat, the women's branch of the Histadrut labor organization, is one of the most impressive women's organizations in the world) and at the local level in, for instance, school and building committees. For many Israeli women, formal and informal support mechanisms are already in place and available to be nurtured and built upon as part of a conscious feminist agenda. Meeting in groups not only leads to political savvy but also allows women to share their counter-hegemonic perceptions and intuitions—thus loosening the stranglehold of patriarchal consciousness. Results of this loosening can already be seen, for instance, in the increasingly critical attention that women and women's groups have begun to give to militarism—one of the prime social and political institutions that naturalizes and demands the subordination of women.

The value of motherhood in Jewish and Israeli culture gives women certain symbolic and pragmatic leverage. Motherhood has been evoked as the grounds for legislating significant rights and services for women. From the first years of the state, Israel embraced legislation that makes gender discrimination illegal and passed laws that protect women's rights in certain circumstances. These laws may be underused but they are on the books and can be invoked and enforced, especially by the many young women now filling the classes of Israel's law schools. The presence of what I have called women gatekeepers in key institutions means that potential leaders are strategically positioned to work for the betterment of women's condition. As feminist consciousness spreads, women gatekeepers—supported by women's organizations—may increasingly understand their own absence of authority within male-dominated institutions, and may begin to shift their allegiance in the direction of their women clients rather than their inequitable employers.

While women's *bodies* are construed as problematic in Jewish culture, biblical tradition lauds heroines who attained their own goals or who saved the Jewish people through their *words*, whether poetry (Deborah), prayer (Hannah), cunning (Miriam), trickery (Judith), persuasion (Esther), insistence (daughters of Zelofhad), or complaining (Rachel).[6] In contemporary Israel, the willingness and ability of women to speak out continues to serve them well. Sima, Zehava, Sarah, Mazal and Rachel—the women whose voices we heard on the first page of this book—have done their part by resolutely drawing attention to the sickening corporeal consequences of the iniquities and inequities of patriarchy. I look forward to seeing their granddaughters find methods of resistance that will acknowledge the pernicious cultural basis to women's illness, and that will allow them to move on to lives of health, strength, and power.

Notes

Introduction: The Cultural Politics of Somatization (1–18)

1. Jewish Israeli women's "survival advantage" is 3.6 years. Arab Israeli women outlive Arab Israeli men by only 1.5 years, which is one quarter of the survival advantage of European women.

2. The women who filled out the questionnaire were fairly representative of Israeli women in terms of age, family income, education, employment status, number of children, and other key demographic indicators.

3. Among young and middle-aged Israelis, men are more likely than women to be admitted to psychiatric hospitals. At age sixty-five and over the trend is reversed, and hospitalization rates for women are 40% higher than for men (cited in Ifrah 1999, 139). A comparison of age-specific suicide rates among women in the United States and Israel reveals much higher suicide rates in Israel for women over age sixty-five, while among men suicide rates are considerably higher in the United States in all adult age groups (cited in Ifrah 1999, 152–153).

4. In various cultures, nervousness, childlessness, depression, diarrhea, diaper rash, allergies, runny noses, benign growths in the breast, menopause, anger, drunkenness, sexual promiscuity, disinterest in sexuality, aging, pain, fatigue, delicacy, corpulence, stress, or headaches are considered illnesses and the people whose bodies bear or wear these conditions are considered ill. In other cultures some or none of these conditions are considered illnesses, and people whose bodies bear or wear these conditions are considered perfectly normal and healthy. Likewise, in some cultures, character traits such as aggression or passivity are considered "natural" to men or to women and even explained in terms of such physiological factors as hormones, while in other cultures the same traits may be considered idiosyncratic, desirable for everyone, or undesirable for everyone regardless of gender.

5. Race and age are other cultural constructs that fit the model I suggest here.

6. A desert fruit that is prickly on the outside but sweet on the inside, the *sabra* was a symbol of the new generation of Israelis.

7. Even among those who self-define as totally nonobservant, most do observe some aspects of traditional Judaism (such as attending a Passover seder and lighting

Chanuka candles). Elihu Katz, one of the authors of the study, clarifies some of the findings of this already classic account of Israeli Jewish religiosity.

> On the basis of these data one can conclude that (a) observance, while partial and selective, is not random, individual, and unsystematic; there is a pattern of practice that describes the (religious) behavior of Jewish Israelis; (b) these observances are not without intent; they may lack "proper" intent but they are motivated by a conscious commitment to the continuity of the Jewish people; (c) moreover, those who observe them are not without belief; religious faith is widespread and there is a high correlation between ritual performance and belief; (d) the most observant group (25–30%) and the rest differ at the level of acceptance of the authority that dictates practice; and a majority of those who practice are apparently aware of the "deviations" and are unperturbed by them, even if many would opt to be "more religious" than they are at the present. (1997, 82–83)

8. As in other countries, mortality rates after acute myocardial infarction and following coronary bypass surgery in Israel are higher among women than men. The factors that may explain this excess mortality include the older age of women patients, their smaller body size, more frequent coexisting illnesses, delay in diagnosis and treatment, and poorer health care (Ifrah 1999, 88).

9. In India, for example, when the rate of women's workforce participation increases, their survival rates improve (Waldron 1991, 31). This may reflect families' willingness to invest more in girls and women who produce income, and it may be a consequence of women's having more say (as income earners) over how the money is spent.

10. Responsibility is of course the central theme in Jewish religious observance; the whole system of *mitzvot* (commandments) has to do with one's responsibilities to God and to other humans.

11. Leah Shakdiel beautifully sums up the experience of Israeli women as "driving full gas in neutral" (personal communication).

12. The implications of women's exclusion from positions of power within he health care system can be serious. Herceptin, a drug that can offer substantial life-enhancing and life-prolonging benefits to women suffering from a certain type of breast cancer, was excluded from the "basket of services" authorized by Israel's Ministry of Health in 1999. Haim Shadmi, a reporter from *HaAretz* obtained a transcript of the session at which the Ministry's Committee—composed almost entirely of men—discussed the matter. Most of the discussion centered on the cost of providing patients with the medication, with few participants expressing any noticeable respect or regard for women's health needs and rights. The most extreme comments were made by Professor Mordechai Shani, director-general of Tel Hashomer Hospital, who explained his opposition to authorizing Herceptin in this way: "We have to be careful about making decisions for a small group in an hysterical situation. I am quite clear on the sensitivity of the breast. I am also quite clear on the sensitivity of everybody else" (*HaAretz* October 19, 1999).

1. Collective Representations of Motherhood (23–38)

1. Israel is not the only country in which women's reproduction is drafted into the service of the state, nor is it the only country in which religious discourse overlays demographic policy. Obermeyer argues that economic pressures and political expediency played a considerable role in Iran's fluctuating population policies, and

each change in policy was justified using religious ideology and selective references to Islamic tradition (Obermeyer 1994).

2. Unless noted otherwise, all quotations of Knesset members are my translations from the Knesset protocols.

3. Policies of this sort are not unique to Israel. Certain other Western countries have also taken measures of various sorts to encourage hospital births.

4. On August 2, 1954, some of the same issues came up again during the second and third readings of the Women's Labor Law. These discussions centered on the matter of maternity leave in the case of miscarriage or stillbirth. The Knesset proceedings preserve a record of a large group of men (more or less informed about the physiology of childbirth) discussing the status of women's bodies. The majority opinion seems to have been that a woman should not receive maternity leave after a miscarriage but should receive it after a stillbirth. Knesset members proposed that if a woman wishes to return to work after a stillbirth, she first must receive permission from a doctor. They discussed limitations on work from the fifth or sixth month of pregnancy, what kinds of work should be forbidden to women, and who should have the authority to decide these matters—the minister of labor or the minister together with the labor unions. Typically, no mention was made of women's having the right or the knowledge to decide for themselves.

5. A paraphrase of Genesis 1:28.

6. See chapter 2, note 13.

7. The entire conceptual basis of Israel's abortion law and abortion debate is different from the American law. The American law considers the status of the fetus—at what point it is considered a human being. The Israeli law considers the circumstances under which the pregnancy occurred. This contrast is rooted partially in differences between Christian (especially Catholic) and Jewish beliefs and law.

8. None of these pamphlets has a year or place of publication printed on them. They are written and privately printed by Efrat.

2. The Reproductive Body (42–66)

1. Misgav Ladach has been, and continues to be, the pioneering Israeli hospital in allowing women some control over their own childbirth experiences. Any critical comments made in this chapter regarding the way childbirth is managed in Israel apply equally—or even to a greater degree—to other Israeli hospitals as well as to Misgav Ladach.

2. The underrepresentation of secular, Ashkenazi Jews is a reflection of Jerusalem demographics; the overrepresentation of American-born women is a consequence of their greater acquaintance with natural childbirth ideologies and their greater inclination to choose Misgav Ladach Hospital because they like its practices.

3. Israeli hospitals did not make available to me statistics on the rate of caesarian sections. According to a study conducted in 1995, the rate of c-sections at Israeli hospitals ranged from 6% to 24% (Zalcberg et al. 1999, 9).

4. Much of what I found in my study is comparable to the findings of Robbie Davis-Floyd (1992) in the United States, especially her observations on how hospital rituals reflect and reinforce the core values of the culture and on their power to shape the experiences and sense of self of birthing women.

5. There are some midwives who spend a great deal of time with each woman, and who patiently and affectionately coach them through labor and delivery. Misgav

Ladach employs an exceptional number of midwives of this sort. The norm throughout Israel, however, is as I have described in this chapter.

6. In a study conducted in Israel in 1995, postpartum women reported greater satisfaction with physicians than with midwives or ward nurses, although in most births the physician is scarcely present either during labor or on the ward after the birth (Zalcberg et al. 1999, 27).

7. All names of postpartum women and midwives are pseudonyms.

8. I use the word "folk" with some reluctance to describe traditional beliefs and practices that are not required by Jewish law or sacralized by wide prescription in sacred texts.

9. I have not included in this list rituals aimed at promoting conception performed by women who feel or felt themselves to be infertile. Because infertility is understood by Israeli women to be an illness and/or a punishment from God, while pregnancy is understood to be healthy and a gift from God (even when there are complications), the two sets of rituals demand separate analyses.

10. I assume to weigh and clean her.

11. Note that in Jewish tradition Eve gave Adam a nameless fruit, not an apple. The apple tradition is a Christian one, but has widely infiltrated Jewish folk beliefs.

12. The National Registry of the Israeli Association for Fertility Research reported in 1992 that 23.6% of IVF deliveries between 1982 and 1989 were multiple births, and 28.6% were preterm. Perinatal mortality rates were 22.8 per 1,000 live births, which was double the ratio found in the general population (cited in Ifrah 1999, 44).

13. Success rates vary from clinic to clinic depending upon the skill and technology of the particular clinic, the way the clinic calculates success rates (conception, carrying pregnancy to term), and whether (or the extent to which) the clinic prescreens in order to select likely candidates. Lauri Pasch and Christine Dunkel-Schetter found an average success rate for IVF of about 15% per treatment cycle (that is, ovary stimulation, egg retrieval, fertilization, transfer). Studies show that people using IVF and other technologies tend to overestimate their chances of success, leading to an emotional rollercoaster.

14. As Leah Shakdiel has pointed out, women are considered defective when infertile, while men are considered defective when incapable of sex (defined in a rather limited, culture-specific manner)—hence the recent Israeli policy that health insurance pays partially for Viagra but not for contraception.

15. Thanks to Gail Labovitz for bringing this text to my attention.

16. There was one group of women in the study who consistently expressed confidence in their ability to breastfeed. When I asked about their plans to breastfeed, the American born women all answered clearly "yes," with the exception of one woman who answered with an equally clear "no."

17. These interviews were carried out by Yvonne Deutsch.

18. This sort of ambivalence regarding women's breasts reiterates in the discourse and practices of breast cancer and breast cancer treatment in Israel (see Sered and Tabory 1999).

3. The Militarized Body (68–103)

1. This term is taken from Yuval-Davis (1985, 654).

2. The cultural construction of women as victims develops rapidly over the Israeli

life cycle: In one major study it was found that while boys were slightly overrepresented among very young children presenting to emergency rooms as a consequence of violence, in the six-to-fourteen age group, 55% of victims were girls, and among adolescents, girls predominated as victims in almost all categories of physical and sexual abuse (cited in Ifrah 1999, 166–167).

3. The social reinforcement that Israeli girls receive for being nice and amiable does not serve them well in a society in which aggression is valued and even valorized (I thank Leah Shakdiel for pointing this out to me).

4. In a study of parental reaction to the draft of their eldest son into the IDF, mothers were found to rate significantly higher than fathers on emotional investment (longing for the son, anxiety about his safety and well-being, preoccupation with his absence and leaves, desire to indulge the son, and various concerns about him). In contrast, fathers scored higher on the belief in military service fostering a son's maturity (the extent to which military service is regarded as advancing the son to a more mature development phase in his life). Generally, the gender differences indicate a more intense and demanding challenge on the mothers' part" (Lomranz et al. 1996, 168).

5. Run by the Center for Parenting and Families in the Community in coordination with the Education Ministry.

6. My claim that war makes Israeli women sick has been backed up by "hard" evidence. Rofe and Goldberg (1983) found that both during the Yom Kippur War and during the relatively calm period preceding it, pregnant women who lived in higher stress environments (nearer to active borders) had higher blood pressure than women who lived in lower stress environments. Lomranz et al. (1994) found that women more than men experienced marked increases in depressive moods during the SCUD missile attacks of the Gulf War, although there was not a significant gender difference in depression before or after the attacks.

7. I have taught a course on anthropology of gender for over a decade. The students consistently find the issue of women in military service especially engaging, and I typically receive several research papers on the topic each year. I have used the framework of classes dealing with gender attended by post–military service young women as opportunities to lead guided discussions about their own experiences in the IDF.

8. On the one hand, Orna Sasson-Levy has pointed out to me that the IDF is less of a total institution than some other armies, since IDF soldiers do stay in close contact with their homes and families. On the other hand, as in all armies, IDF soldiers can only go home when given leave, and thus their contact with family and home is mediated by IDF policy which varies among units, commanding officers, and over time. Moreover, it is often the case that the family reinforces IDF culture, both because the young man's father and other male relatives have served in the IDF and because families are expected by the IDF to support their sons in various ways during their service.

9. Young women who become pregnant during their required service in the IDF are officially ineligible to continue serving. Women who decide to terminate the pregnancy are offered a document to sign volunteering to continue their service. A second pregnancy may be met with less support from the IDF. It seems that repeated pregnancies during IDF service are most common among young women from disadvantaged backgrounds who may not have the financial means to purchase contraception. Birth control is not provided by the IDF, and salaries of soldiers during the years of required service are very low.

10. This is custom, not law.

11. Orna Sasson-Levy clarifies that the IDF does not treat women soldiers or women soldiers' bodies in a unified way. There is a great deal of variation depending upon the soldier's role, base, area in the country, and so on (personal communication).

12. Orna Sasson-Levy has pointed out to me that the basic training of noncombatant men also emphasizes developing an orderly and controlled body (but not a pleasant body). She has also found that men in noncombat positions often gain weight and lose physical fitness throughout their service.

13. The slogan "The best [men] to pilot school" was used as a recruitment advertisement. Weizman's addition seems almost inevitable.

14. Perhaps the most ironic twist on the public construction of women soldiers as victims can be found in incidents in which an Arab passerby rescues a Jewish woman soldier from a Jewish rapist (see, for example, the *Jerusalem Post*, June 26, 1991). This sort of scenario blurs gender and national hierarchies, and presents women soldiers as so terribly vulnerable that even "the enemy" takes pity on them.

15. Tuten notes that during World War II the Germans did not let their servicewomen use weapons even in self-defense (1982, 243).

16. Nira Yuval-Davis (1997) makes the important point that in colonial situations men are defined as effeminate; thus liberation movements often include a strong macho dimension. One can easily see that this analysis fits well the Jewish transition from the diaspora to building the Zionist state. The "New Jew" was conceived as strong, brave, and very masculine.

17. There are anecdotal reports of women soldiers who complained of harassment and were then transferred (against their wishes) to other units. Apparently, this is done when the harassing officer is considered more important than the harassed soldier to the functioning of the unit. There are also reports that it is not uncommon for co-workers to ostracize women soldiers who complain of harassment.

18. Men who sexually harass women within the IDF are usually tried and punished within the framework of the IDF rather than in civil court. Thus a first-class sergeant major who made a practice of pinching the buttocks of women soldiers at his base was demoted to sergeant major and given a two-month suspended sentence by a Haifa military court. The military judges noted that in sentencing the officer they "took an extremely grave view of his actions" (*Jerusalem Post*, September 21, 1992), yet for reasons unclear to me did not discharge him from the IDF or send him to prison.

19. According to the Association of Rape Crisis Centers in Israel, only about 15% of rapes are reported either to the police or to a rape crisis center (personal communication, 1999).

20. Orna Sasson-Levy tells me that one year later the school staff talks about the rape in terms of "the incident," "the event," "the thing that happened," consistently avoiding the word *rape*.

21. Among the women interviewed, the lifetime rate of crime victimization was 57%. Koss measured levels of victimization using a scale escalating from never victimized, to victim of mild (non-contact) crimes, victim of bodily harm but not rape, serious victimization including rape, and finally victim of multiple assaults including rape.

4. The Ritualized Body (105–121)

1. Given the intimate emotional and geographic relationships between men and women in most cultures, symbolic rather than overtly violent means are usually the preferred means for structuring heterosexual society.

2. During the time in which the Temple was the focus of Jewish life, menstruation precluded involvement in Temple worship. At the end of the seven-day period of impurity, women were required to bring a sacrifice to the Temple, before resuming participation in Temple ritual.

3. Levi, Levinsohn, and Katz (1993) report that 24% of Jewish Israeli women go to the mikveh (16% regularly and 8% occasionally). This figure however does not seem to be controlled to exclude women who do not menstruate because of age or because of continuous cycles of pregnancy and lactation.

4. Levi, Levinsohn, and Katz (1993) number this group, depending on the measure, at between 7% and 20% of the Jewish population.

5. I suspect that this differs from Ashkenazi women in the United States.

6. Their mothers and grandmothers were more religiously observant, but most are now postmenopausal and so rarely have reason to come to the mikveh.

7. I suspect they are referring to Bela Schick, who developed a test for diphtheria antibodies.

8. I have made an informal study of mikveh booklets in the United States. While there is some overlap (booklets put out by the Lubavitcher movement, for example, are published in both Hebrew and English), my sense is that booklets emphasizing miraculous healing and other miracles are more popular in Israel than in the United States.

9. In mikvehs in the United States it is not uncommon to find breast self-examination guides hung up in each room for the convenience of mikveh patrons. The pattern I am describing in this chapter represents the particularly Israeli playing-out of Jewish themes, which is not the only way that these themes can be or are played-out.

10. In Jewish cultures, women's bodies often are understood to be sources of pollution, while men's bodies are seen as sources of blessing (rabbis hold up their hands in blessing as do priests, and some put their hands on heads of people to bless them; physical contact with tombs of saints is believed to spread blessings, and almost all holy tombs are of male saints).

11. In public life, gender differences were significant: Women were excluded from the world of learning and from roles of community leadership (see Wegner 1988, 75 ff.).

12. I suspect that members of the Knesset have little knowledge or concern for what goes on in the mikvehs. The coercive nature of prenuptial mikveh rituals is a "minor" by-product of the law that gives religious authorities (Jewish, Christian, and Muslim) a monopoly over marriage and divorce in Israel.

13. I thank my student Marilyn Froggatt (Hebrew University, 1998) for pointing out to me some of the more interesting elements of the *bedeken* ceremony.

14. The ethnography on which this section is based was collected during systematic observations of brides' visits to the mikveh over a period of four months at one mikveh in Jerusalem, and twenty years of less systematic observations.

15. These three commandments often are grouped together as the paradigmatic women's commandments. It is written in the Mishnah that women die in childbirth as a result of neglecting these commandments (see the epigraph at the beginning of this chapter).

5. The Scrutinized Body (124–151)

1. At age eleven, Israeli girls rank the highest of twenty-three European countries in television watching, and Israeli boys rank second. By age thirteen Israeli boys move down to seventh place, where they remain through age fifteen, while Israeli

girls continue to top the list, beat only marginally by Welsh girls and boys (Harel, Kaneh, and Rahav 1997, 129).

2. This particular list was compiled by Carl Alpert, one of my favorite observers of Israeli society, and printed in the *Jewish Advocate* in September 1999. In a similar vein, at a 1999 ceremony held at the President's House in honor of schools that had excelled at soliciting donations to charity, *all* of the dignitaries who spoke on behalf of the state and the education system (with the exception of the wife of the President, Mrs. Reuma Weizman) were men. The charitable organizations that benefitted from the schools' efforts, on the other hand, were represented by three young women, each of whom was a sufferer of a physical or social disability.

3. For example, Amram (1992) shows an advertisement for Johnson's baby oil in which the 1978 Israeli version does not expose the model's face while the English language version does.

4. In a seamless mixture of the medical establishment and the marketplace, the exhibit was sponsored by companies that make baby equipment and by a magazine called *Pregnancy and Baby*, and was held "under the patronage" of Professor Mark Glazerman of Wolfson Medical Center, Professor Shlomo Mashiach, director of the obstetrics/gynecology department of Shiba Medical Center, and Dr. Michael Stark, medical director of Misgav Ladach Hospital.

5. A similar advertisement reads: "Passover Special for 1998 for members of the Maccabi, Leumit and Meuhedet Health Funds: Members can join the thousands of satisfied people who have had operations all over the country and enjoy the unprecedentedly low prices found only at the largest clinic for aesthetic surgery. Call now." The advertisement offers breast augmentation and reduction, fat suctioning, hair removal, hair transplants, and so on.

6. This data was drawn from reports of breast-implant importers.

7. Rosenblum makes references to, and rumors circulate about, her alleged love affairs with Edward Kennedy, Robert DeNiro, and Salvador Dali.

8. Rosenblum acknowledges that her style and language are similar to Eva Peron's.

9. Women were in slots 4, 5, 9, 10; men in slots 1, 2, 3, 6, 7, 8. To be fair, Meretz has by far the largest proporrtion of women in the Knesset of all major parties.

10. Recently there has been some shift toward more favorable public opinion.

11. Bonna Deborah Haberman, an active member of Women of the Wall who has written and spoken extensively about the case, tells me that there has been a development in the responses to the Women of the Wall over the years. While in the beginning the Women were subjected to some rather nasty curses (for example, "You should never have children!"), some later responses have been more subtle and intellectually engaged.

12. A second category of invectives plugs into the cultural understanding that black clothing is worn by mourners. "I hope you wear black all you life" and "I hope your son dies and you won't be able to visit his grave" (Helman and Rapoport 1997, 690–691) are curses that remind women of their impotence to protect their sons in militarized societies, and even suggest that women's protest may (in either a political or supernatural way) cause men to die at war.

13. The anecdotes cited in this section are a small sample of dozens of similar modesty demands recently reported in the press. In order to avoid making this chapter unwieldy, I have not cited multiple newspaper references to the same issue, but the interested reader can consult other newspapers of the same day or week in order to learn more about the issues. Wherever possible, I cite the *Jerusalem Post* so that the references will be accessible to English-language readers.

14. After women members of the moshav protested, the elders came up with a

different reason for the disasters: that the swimming pool was open on the Sabbath and holidays.

15. These are rallies in which rabbis and other Orthodox speakers urge secular Jews to "return" to Orthodox Judaism and urge Orthodox Jews to deepen their faith and commitment.

16. An event of this sort held on December 3, 1997, at Yad Eliahu was attended by ten thousand women, most wearing "secular" clothes.

17. According to Orthodox Jewish law, married women must cover their hair for reasons of modesty. The "problem" with wigs is that, unlike scarves or hats, wigs can look like the wearer's own hair, and so some rabbis judge them to be insufficient as hair coverings.

18. 1 Kings 11:25 ff.

19. Taking the opposite view, one of the largest Ashkenazi ultra-Orthodox sects, Chabad (Lubavitch), strongly urges women to wear wigs rather than scarves. The reasoning is that scarves accidentally can slip off the head, too easily can be taken off and put in one's purse when the mood strikes, and are so light and comfortable that the woman can forget she is wearing it and behave in a manner inappropriate for a pious, married Jewish woman.

20. The gap between the Israeli girls and girls in the next highest ranking society, French Belgium, begins at 2% at age eleven, reaching 10% in the mid-teenage years (Harel, Kaneh, and Rahav 1997, 122). Let me add as a caveat that epidemics of eating disorders tend to follow in the paths of other cultural changes which reach various countries at varying speeds, suggesting that differences in rates of eating disorders could be blips on the chart that will tend to even out over a period of years.

21. In this study, in all of the measures of dieting (use of diet pills, vomiting, laxatives, and doctors' supervision), Arab girls significantly outranked Jewish girls (Harel, Kaneh, and Rahav 1997).

Conclusion: Resisting Bodies (155–170)

1. I thank Deborah Greniman for bringing this passage to my attention.

2. There certainly are some mikveh attendants who help their women clients conceptualize their own bodies, their relationships with their husband, and even their notions of God and Jewish law in radically liberating ways. I have written about one such attendant in Sered 1997a. But these sorts of mikveh attendants are few and far between.

3. At the same time, the women who encounter these gatekeepers usually do know, at some level, where the true authority lies. Both mikveh attendants and midwives make continuous references to the expert opinions of the men who are "over" them.

4. In order to protect my informants, I will not spell out the techniques used.

5. The founding of Parents Against Silence can be dated to an open letter published in Israeli newspapers on April 26 and 27, 1983. Written by Shoshana Shmueli, the mother of a soldier serving in Lebanon, the letter was a collective declaration of parental guilt for having raised children to believe that militarism is a national virtue.

6. Deborah (Judges 5:1), Hannah (1 Samuel 1:10–11), Miriam (Exodus 2:7), Judith (Book of Judith), Esther (Book of Esther), Rachel (Genesis 30:1), daughters of Zelofhad (Numbers 27:1–11).

Works Cited

Abu-Lughod, Lila. 1990. "The Romance of Resistance: Tracing Transformations of Power through Bedouin Women." *American Ethnologist* 17: 41–55.

Adler, Nancy E., and Marilee Coriell. 1997. "Socioeconomic Status and Women's Health." In *Health Care for Women: Psychological, Social, and Behavioral Influences*, edited by Sheryle J. Gallant, Gwendolyn Puryear Keita, and Renee Royak-Schaler, 11–24. Washington, D.C.: American Psychological Association.

Amir, Delila. 1995. "Responsible, Committed and Wise: The Establishment of Israeli Femininity in Committees to Terminate Pregnancy." *Teoria VeBikoret* 7: 247–254.

Amir, Delila, and Orly Biniamin. 1992. "Abortion Approval as a Ritual of Symbolic Control. In *The Criminalization of a Woman's Body*, edited by Clarice Feinman, 5–25. New York: Haworth Press.

———. 1997. "Defining Encounters: Who Are the Women Entitled to Join the Israeli Collective." *Women's Studies International Forum* 20 (5/6): 639–650.

Amram, Meirav. 1992. "Female Stereotypes in Advertisements in Israel Between 1974 and 1989." Unpublished paper.

Apter, Alan, Mohammed Abu Shah, Iulian Iancu, Henry Abramovitch, Abraham Weizman, and Samuel Tyano. 1994. "Cultural Effects on Eating Attitudes in Israeli Subpopulations and Hospitalized Anorectics." *Genetic, Social, and General Psychology Monographs* 120 (1): 83–99.

Arian, Asher, Ilan Talmud, and Tamar Hermann. 1988. *National Security and Public Opinion in Israel*. Boulder, Colo.: Westview Press (published for the Jaffee Center for Strategic Studies, Tel Aviv University).

Ariel, Mira. 1988. "Female and Male Stereotypes in Israeli Literature and Media: Evidence from Introductory Patterns." *Language and Communication* 8 (1): 43–68.

Avgar, Amy. 1997. "Women's Health in Israel: A Feminist Perspective." *Social Work in Health Care* 25 (1/2): 45–62.

Avgar, Amy, and Carol Gordon. 1997. "Your Health: Results and Conclusions" (in Hebrew). *At* 62–65.

Avorva, Miriam, Ziona Haklai, Hava Klein, and Meir Handelsman. 1996. *Health in Israel: Selected Statistics*. Israel Ministry of Health.

Baider, Leah. 1996. "Emotional Characteristics of Women with Breast Cancer." In *Breast Cancer in Israel*, edited by Amy Avgar, 131–137. Jerusalem: Brookdale Institute.

Bar-Yosef, Rivka, and Dorit Padan-Eisenstark. 1977. "Role System Under Stress: Sex Roles in War." *Social Problems* 25: 135–144.

Barnoy, Zipi. 1997. "The IDF Women's Corps as Seen by the Written Press and by Its Commanding Officers, 1948–1996." Master's thesis, Bar Ilan University.

Ben-Ari, Eyal. 1998. *Mastering Soldiers: Conflict, Emotion and the Enemy in an Israeli Military Unit*. New York: Berghahn Books.

Ben-Zur, Hasida, and Moshe Zeidner. 1996. "Gender Differences in Coping Reactions under Community Crisis and Daily Routine Conditions." *Personality and Individual Differences* 20 (3): 331–340.

Berkovitch, Nitza. 1997. "Motherhood as a National Mission: The Construction of Womanhood in the Legal Discourse in Israel." *Women's Studies International Forum* 20 (5/6): 605–619.

Bloom, Anne R. 1993. "Women in the Defense Forces." In *Calling the Equality Bluff: Women in Israel*, edited by Barbara Swirski and Marilyn Safir, 128–138. New York and London: Teachers College Press.

Bolin, Anne. 1992. "Vandalized Vanity: Feminine Physiques Betrayed and Portrayed." In *Tattoo, Torture, Mutilation, and Adornment: The Denaturalization of the Body in Culture and Text*, edited by Frances E. Mascia-Lees and Patricia Sharpe, 79–99. Albany: State University of New York Press.

Bornstein, Galit, and Zofit Ben-Ari. 1997. "The Presentation of Women and Men as They are Reflected in Advertisements in Israeli Newspapers." Unpublished paper.

Boyarin, Daniel. 1997. *Unheroic Conduct: The Rise of Heterosexuality and the Invention of the Jewish Man*. Berkeley: University of California Press.

Brodie, Janine. 1994. "Health versus Rights: Comparative Perspectives on Abortion Policy in Canada and the United States." In *Power and Decision: The Social Control of Reproduction*, edited by Gita Sen and Rachel C. Snow, 123–146. Boston: Harvard School of Public Health and Harvard University Press.

Brownmiller, Susan. 1975. *Against Our Will: Men, Women and Rape*. New York: Simon and Schuster.

Bruch, Hilde. 1978. *The Golden Cage: The Enigma of Anorexia Nervosa*. Cambridge: Harvard University Press.

Chesney, Margaret A. 1991. "Women, Work-Related Stress, and Smoking." In *Women, Work, and Health: Stress and Opportunities*, edited by Marianne Frankenhaeuser, Ulf Lundberg, and Margaret Chesney, 139–155. New York and London: Plenum Press.

Chill, Abraham. 1989. *The Minhagim*. New York: Sepher-Hermon Press.

Cicurel, Inbal Esther. n.d. "The Rabbinate Versus Jewish Women: The Mikvah as a Contested Domain." Unpublished manuscript.

———. 1998. "The Mikvah—Why Do They Use It? Female Views and Uses of the Jewish Ritual Bath." Master's thesis, Ben Gurion University, Department of Sociology and Anthropology.

Coleman, Linda, and Cindy Dickinson. 1984. "The Risks of Healing: The Hazards of the Nursing Profession." In *Double Exposure: Women's Health Hazards on the Job and at Home*, edited by Wendy Chavkin, 37–56. New York: Monthly Review Press.

Condit, Celeste Michelle. 1990. *Decoding Abortion Rhetoric: Communicating Social Change*. Urbana and Chicago: University of Illinois Press.

Crisp, A. H. [1980] 1995. *Anorexia Nervosa: Let Me Be*. Hove, England: Lawrence Erlbaum.

Crull, Peggy. 1984. "Sexual Harassment and Women's Health." In *Double Exposure: Women's Health Hazards on the Job and at Home*, edited by Wendy Chavkin, 100–120. New York: Monthly Review Press.

Daly, Mary. 1978. *Gyn/Ecology*. Boston: Beacon Press.

Datan, Nancy, Aaron Antonovsky, and Benjamin Maoz. 1981. *A Time to Reap: The Middle Age of Women in Five Israeli Subcultures*. Baltimore: Johns Hopkins University Press.

Davis, Kathy, and Sue Fisher. 1993. "Power and the Female Subject." In *Negotiating at the Margins: The Gendered Discourses of Power and Resistance*, edited by Sue Fisher and Kathy Davis, 3–20. New Brunswick, N.J.: Rutgers University Press.

Davis-Floyd, Robbie E. 1992. *Birth as an American Rite of Passage*. Berkeley: University of California Press.

Deutsch, Yvonne. 1994. "Israeli Women against the Occupation: Political Growth and the Persistence of Ideology." Translated by Andre Rosenthal. In *Women and the Israeli Occupation: The Politics of Change*, edited by Tamar Mayer, 88–104. London: Routledge.

Douglas, Mary. 1975. *Implicit Meanings*. London: Routledge and Kegan Paul.

———. 1982. *Natural Symbols*. New York: Pantheon Books.

Doyal, Lesley. 1995. *What Makes Women Sick: Gender and the Political Economy of Health*. New Brunswick, N.J.: Rutgers University Press.

Dyregrov, Atle, and Stig Berge Matthieson. 1987. "Similarities and Differences in Mothers' and Fathers' Grief Following the Death of an Infant." *Scandinavian Journal of Psychology* 28 (1): 1–15.

El-Or, Tamar, and Gideon Aran. 1995. "Giving Birth to a Settlement: Maternal Thinking and Political Action of Jewish Women on the West Bank." *Gender and Society* 9: 60–78.

Enloe, Cynthia. 1983. *Does Khaki Become You?: The Militarization of Women's Lives*. Boston: South End Press.

Eshed, Hana. 1991. "Morbidity Factors among Women: Research Findings." In *Women's Health in Israel*, edited by Amy Avgar, 35–40. Jerusalem: Israel Women's Network.

Ettinger, Amos. 1993. *Quarter Before Joining the Army*. Ramat Gan, Israel: Avivim.

Finkler, Kaja. 1994. *Women in Pain: Gender and Morbidity in Mexico*. Philadelphia: University of Pennsylvania Press.

First, Anat. 1981. "Sexual Representation and Sexual Stereotypes as Reflected in Advertisements in Israeli Newspapers." Master's thesis, Tel Aviv University.

———. 1998. "Nothing New Under the Sun? A Comparison of Images of Women in Israeli Advertisements in 1979 and 1994." *Sex Roles* 38 (11/12): 1065–1077.

Foucault, Michel. 1977. *Discipline and Punish: The Birth of the Prison*. London: Tavistock.

———. 1980. *The History of Sexuality: An Introduction*. New York: Vintage.

Frankenhaeuser, Marianne. 1991. "The Psychophysiology of Sex Differences as Related to Occupational Stress." In *Women, Work, and Health: Stress and Opportunities*, edited by Marianne Frankenhaeuser, Ulf Lundberg, and Margaret Chesney, 39–61. New York and London: Plenum Press.

Geertz, Clifford. 1973. *The Interpretation of Cultures*. New York: Basic Books.

Gilat, Nurit. 1987. "The Roaring Silence: Parents Against Silence." Master's thesis, Haifa University, Department of Political Science.

Ginzberg, Louis. 1947. *The Legends of the Jews*. Translated from the German by Henrietta Szold. Philadelphia: Jewish Publication Society of America.

Goffman, Erving. 1962. *Asylums: Essays on the Social Situation of Mental Patients and Other Inmates*. Chicago: Aldine.

Golan, Galia. 1997. "Militarization and Gender: The Israeli Experience." *Women's Studies International Forum* 20 (5/6): 581–586.

Golden, Stephanie. 1998. *Slaying the Mermaid: Women and the Culture of Sacrifice*. New York: Harmony Books.

Goldman, Nancy Loring, editor. 1982. *Female Soldiers—Combatants or Noncombatants?: Historical and Contemporary Perspectives*. Westport, Conn.: Greenwood Press.

Gordon, Richard A. 1990. *Anorexia and Bulimia: Anatomy of a Social Epidemic*. Cambridge, Mass.: B. Blackwell.

Griffin, Susan. [1979] 1986. *Rape: The Politics of Consciousness*. San Francisco: Harper and Row.

Grosz, Elizabeth. 1993. "Bodies and Knowledge: Feminism and the Crisis of Reason." In *Feminist Epistemologies*, edited by Linda Alcoff and Elizabeth Potter, 187–216. New York: Routledge.

Guillaumin, Colette. 1993. "The Constructed Body." Translated by Diane Griffin Crowder. In *Reading the Social Body*, edited by Catherine B. Burroughs and Jeffrey David Ehrenreich, 40–60. Iowa City: University of Iowa Press.

Haas, Danielle. 1999. "When the Woman of Valor Has Anorexia." *Jerusalem Report*, July 5.

Handwerker, Lisa. 1998. "The Consequences of Modernity for Childless Women in China: Medicalization and Resistance." In *Pragmatic Women and Body Politics*, edited by Margaret Lock and Patricia A. Kaufert, 178–205. Cambridge: Cambridge University Press.

Hanik, Mira. 1998. *Tipus Nashi: Israeli Career Women Tell of the Path to Success*. Tel Aviv: Sifriat HaMercaz HaYisraeli LeNihul.

Harel, Yossi. 1999. Violence among Youth in Israel 1994–1998: Findings from the National Study on Youth Risk Behaviors and Injuries, World Health Organization Health Behaviors in School-Aged Children. Jerusalem: Bar Ilan University and JDC-Brookdale Institute.

Harel, Yossi, Dafna Kaneh, and Giora Rahav. 1997. *Youth in Israel: Social Welfare, Health, and Risk Behavior from an International Perspective*. Jerusalem: JDC-Brookdale Institute.

Haynes, Suzanne G. 1991. "The Effect of Job Demands, Job Control, and New Technologies on the Health of Employed Women." In *Women, Work, and Health: Stress and Opportunities*, edited by Marianne Frankenhaeuser, Ulf Lundberg, and Margaret Chesney, 157–169. New York and London: Plenum Press.

Hazleton, Lesley. 1977. *Israeli Women: The Reality Behind the Myth*. New York: Simon and Schuster.

Heise, Lori L. 1994. "Gender-Based Abuse: The Global Epidemic." In *Reframing Women's Health*, edited by Alice J. Dan, 233–250. Thousand Oaks Calif.: Sage.

Helman, Sara, and Tamar Rapoport. 1997. "Women in Black: Challenging Israel's Gender and Socio-political Orders." *British Journal of Sociology* 48 (4): 681–700.

Hoffman, Eileen. 1995. *Our Health, Our Lives*. New York: Pocket Books.

Hoffman, Eileen, and Amy Avgar. 1998. "Women's Health in Israel and the United States: A Cross-Cultural Perspective." *Journal of Gender-Specific Medicine* 1 (2): 44–51.

Holroyd, Kenneth A., and Gary L. Lipchik. 1997. "Recurrent Headache Disorders." In *Health Care for Women: Psychological, Social, and Behavioral Influences*, edited by Sheryle J. Gallant, Gwendolyn Puryear Keita, and Renee Royak-Schaler, 365–384. Washington, D.C.: American Psychological Association.

Ifrah, Anneke, editor. 1999. *Women's Health in Israel 1999: A Data Book*. Jerusalem: Hadassah, The Women's Zionist Organization of America and Israel Women's Network.

Israel Central Bureau of Statistics. 1996. *Survey of Use of Health Services, 1993*. Special Publications, 1030–1032. Jerusalem.

———. 1998. *Israel's Statistical Yearbook*. Jerusalem.

———. 1998. Survey 25 (1996/7), Survey 39 (1997). *Selected Characteristics of Women Approaching Committees for Pregnancy Termination in Israel, Supplement to the Statistical Yearbook*. Jerusalem.

Israel Center for Disease Control. 1997. *Condition of Health in Israel*. Tel HaShomer.

Izraeli, Dafna N. 1997. "Gendering Military Service in the Israel Defense Forces." *Israel Social Science Research* 12 (1): 129–166.

Jerby, Iris. 1996. *The Double Price: Women's Status and Military Service in Israel*. Tel Aviv: Ramot Publishers, Tel Aviv University.

Kaffman, Mordechai, and Tovah Sadeh. 1989. "Anorexia Nervosa in the Kibbutz: Factors Influencing the Development of a Monoideistic Fixation." *International Journal of Eating Disorders* 8 (1): 33–53.

Kahn, Susan Martha. 1998. "Rabbis and Reproduction: The Uses of New Reproductive Technologies among Ultraorthodox Jews in Israel." Working Paper Series. Waltham Mass.: International Research Institute on Jewish Women, Brandeis University.

Kampf, Ronit. 1996. "Looking for the Cracks in the Wall: The Interaction between Women's Protest Groups and the Israeli Press." *Patuah* March: 4–26.

Kane, Penny. 1991. *Women's Health from Womb to Tomb*. New York: St. Martin's Press.

Karasek, Robert, D. Baker, F. Marxer, A. Ahlblom, and T. Theorell. 1981. "Job Decision Latitude, Job Demands, and Cardiovascular Disease: A Prospective Study of Swedish Men." *American Journal of Public Health* 71 (7): 694–705.

Karasek, Robert, and Tores Theorell. 1990. *Healthy Work: Stress, Productivity, and the Reconstruction of Working Life*. New York: Basic Books.

Katz, Elihu. 1997. "Behavioral and Phenomenological Jewishness." In *The Jewishness of Israelis: Responses to the Guttman Report*, edited by Charles S. Liebman and Elihu Katz, 71–84. Albany: State University of New York Press.

Kaveh, Ayelet. 1998. "Keeping the Purity Laws: A Form of Healing." Seminar paper. Bar Ilan University, Department of Sociology and Anthropology.

Kedem, Peri. 1991. "Dimensions of Jewish Religiosity in Israel." In *Tradition, Conflict, Innovation: Jewishness and Judaism in Contemporary Israel*, edited by Zvi Sobel amd Benjamin Beit-Hallahmi, 251–277. Albany: State University of New York Press.

Kielmann, Karina. 1998. "Barren Ground: Contested Identities of Infertile Women in Pemba, Tanzenia." In *Pragmatic Women and Body Politics*, edited by Margaret Lock and Patricia A. Kaufert, 127–163. Cambridge: Cambridge University Press.

Kleinman, Arthur. 1992. "Pain and Resistance: The Delegitimation and Relegitimation of Local Worlds." In *Pain as Human Experience: An Anthropological*

Perspective, edited by Mary-Jo DelVecchio Good and et al., 169–197. Berkeley: University of California Press.

Koss, Mary P. 1994. "The Negative Impact of Crime Victimization on Women's Health and Medical Use." In *Reframing Women's Health*, edited by Alice J. Dan, 189–200. Thousand Oaks, Calif.: Sage.

Levy, Shlomit, Hanna Levinsohn, and Elihu Katz. 1993. *Beliefs, Observances and Social Interaction among Israeli Jews*. Jerusalem: Louis Guttman Israel Institute of Applied Social Research.

Levy-Schreiber, Edna. 1998. "Heroes and Helpmates: Militarism, Gender, and National Belonging in Israel." Ph.D. diss. University of California, Irvine.

Lewin, Ellen. 1998. "Wives, Mothers and Lesbians: Rethinking Resistance in the United States." In *Pragmatic Women and Body Politics*, edited by Margaret Lock and Patricia A. Kaufert, 164–177. Cambridge: Cambridge University Press.

Liebman, Charles S. 1997. "Cultural Conflict in Israeli Society." In *The Jewishness of Israelis: Responses to the Guttman Report*, edited by Charles S. Liebman and Elihu Katz, 103–118. Albany: State University of New York Press.

Lincoln, Bruce. 1989. *Discourse and the Construction of Society: Comparative Studies of Myth, Ritual, and Classification*. New York and Oxford: Oxford University Press.

———. 1994. *Authority: Construction and Corrosion*. Chicago: University of Chicago Press.

Lipman-Blumen, Jean. 1984. *Gender Roles and Power*. Englewood Cliffs, N.J.: Prentice-Hall.

Lock, Margaret, and Patricia A. Kaufert. 1998. Introduction to *Pragmatic Women and Body Politics*, edited by Margaret Lock and Patricia A. Kaufert, 1–27. Cambridge: Cambridge University Press.

Lomranz, Jacob, Dov Shmotkin, Nitza Eyal, and Yael Zohar. 1996. "Launching Themes in Israeli Fathers and Mothers." *Journal of Adult Development* 3 (3): 159–169.

Lomranz, Jacob, Steven E. Hobfoll, Robert Johnson, Nitza Eyal, and Mina Zemach. 1994. "A Nation's Response to Attack: Israelis' Depressive Reactions to the Gulf War." *Journal of Traumatic Stress* 7 (1): 59–73.

Lorber, Judith. 1979. "Good Patients and Problem Patients: Conformity and Deviance in a General Hospital." In *Patients, Physicians, and Illness*, edited by E. Gartly Jaco, 185–201. New York: Free Press.

———. 1997. *Gender and the Social Construction of Illness*. Thousand Oaks, Calif.: Sage.

Mark, Mordechai, Jonathan Rabinowitz, Stanley Rabinowitz, Bracha Baoni, Isak Babus, and Yehuda L. Danon. 1993. "Brief Treatment of Anorexia Nervosa in Military Personnel." *Hospital and Community Psychiatry* 44 (1): 69–71.

Marmot, M. G., H. Bosma, H. Hemingway, E. Brunner, and S. Stansfeld. 1997. "Contribution of Job Control and Other Risk Factors to Social Variations in Coronary Heart Disease Incidence." *The Lancet* 350 (9073): 235–239.

Martin, Emily. 1987. *The Woman in the Body*. Boston: Beacon Press.

Mascia-Lees, Frances E., and Patricia Sharpe. 1992. "The Marked and the Un(re)marked: Tattoo and Gender in Theory and Practice." In *Tattoo, Torture, Mutilation, and Adornment: The Denaturalization of the Body in Culture and Text*, edited by Frances E. Mascia-Lees and Patricia Sharpe, 145–169. Albany: State University of New York Press.

Meacham, Tirzah. 1989. "Critical Edition of Mishnah Masechet Niddah with Commentaries upon Nusach and Chapters on the Development of the Halacha and on Realia." Ph.D. diss., Hebrew University, Jerusalem.

Morgan, Kathryn Pauly. 1998. "Contested Bodies, Contested Knowledges: Women, Health, and the Politics of Medicalization." In *The Politics of Women's Health: Exploring Agency and Autonomy*, edited by Susan Sherwin and the Feminist Health Care Ethics Research Network, 83–121. Philadelphia: Temple University Press.

Neriya, Rachel. 1983. *To the Daughter of Israel Approaching Marriage*. Kfar HaRoeh: n.p.

———. 1989. *Happy Marriage*. Jerusalem: The National Center for Family Purity in Israel.

O'Halloran, M. Sean. 1993. *Focus on Eating Disorders: A Reference Handbook*. Santa Barbara: ABC-CLIO.

Obermeyer, Carla Makhlouf. 1994. "Religious Doctrine, State Ideology, and Reproductive Options in Islam." In *Power and Decision: The Social Control of Reproduction*, edited by Gita Sen and Rachel C. Snow, 59–76. Boston, Mass.: Harvard School of Public Health and Harvard University Press.

Okinawa Prefectural Office. 1994. *Okinawa Women's Report*. Naha, Okinawa.

Ortner, Sherry. 1996. *Making Gender: The Politics and Erotics of Culture*. Boston: Beacon Press.

Paige, Karen Erickson, and Jeffery M. Paige. 1981. *Politics of Reproductive Ritual*. Berkeley: University of California Press.

Pasch, Lauri A., and Christine Dunkel-Schetter. 1997. "Fertility Problems: Complex Issues Faced by Women and Couples." In *Health Care for Women: Psychological, Social, and Behavioral Influences*, edited by Sheryle J. Gallant, Gwendolyn Puryear Keita, and Renee Royak-Schaler, 187–202. Washington, D.C.: American Psychological Association.

Pike, Kathleen M., and Ruth H. Striegel-Moore. 1997. "Disordered Eating and Eating Disorders." In *Health Care for Women: Psychological, Social, and Behavioral Influences*, edited by Sheryle J. Gallant, Gwendolyn Puryear Keita, and Renee Royak-Schaler, 97–114. Washington, D.C.: American Psychological Association.

Pitanguy, Jacqueline. 1994. "Feminist Politics and Reproductive Rights: The Case of Brazil." In *Power and Decision: The Social Control of Reproduction*, edited by Gita Sen and Rachel C. Snow, 101–122. Boston, Mass.: Harvard School of Public Health and Harvard University Press.

Pliskin, Karen L. 1987. *Silent Boundaries: Cultural Constraints on Sickness and Diagnosis of Iranians in Israel*. New Haven: Yale University Press.

Prell, Riv-Ellen. 1987. "Sacred Categories and Social Relations: The Visibility and Invisibility of Gender in an American Jewish Community." In *Judaism Viewed from Within and from Without*, edited by Harvey E. Goldberg, 171–194. Albany: State University of New York Press.

Pritchard, Jack, and Paul MacDonald. 1980. *Williams Obstetrics* 16th edition. New York: Appleton-Century-Crafts.

Quester, George H. 1982. "The Problem." In *Female Soldiers—Combatants or Noncombatants?: Historical and Contemporary Perspectives*, edited by Nancy Loring Goldman, 217–236. Westport, Conn.: Greenwood Press.

Rein, Natalie. 1980. *Daughters of Rachel: Women in Israel*. Harmondsworth, Middlesex, England: Penguin Books.

Reiss, Nira, editor. 1998. *Women in Israel: Data and Information*. Jerusalem: Israel Women's Network.

Rofe, Yacov, and Joel Goldberg. 1983. "Prolonged Exposure to a War Environment and Its Effects on the Blood Pressure of Pregnant Women." *British Journal of Social Psychology* 22: 305–311.

Rosaldo, Michelle Zimbalist. 1974. "Women, Culture, and Society: A Theoretical Overview." In *Women, Culture, and Society*, edited by Michelle Zimbalist Rosaldo and Louise Lamphere, 17–42. Stanford: Stanford University Press.

Rosenberg, Harriet G. 1984. "The Home is the Workplace: Hazards, Stress, and Pollutants in the Household." In *Double Exposure: Women's Health Hazards on the Job and at Home*, edited by Wendy Chavkin, 219–245. New York: Monthly Review Press.

Ruzek, Sheryl Burt. 1997. "Access, Cost, and Quality of Medial Care: Where Are We Heading?" In *Women's Health: Complexities and Differences*, edited by Sheryl Burt Ruzek, Virginia L. Olesen, and Adele E. Clarke, 183–230. Columbus: Ohio State University Press.

Sacks, Karen. 1979. *Sisters and Wives*. Westport, Conn.: Greenwood Press.

Said, Edward W. 1978. *Orientalism*. New York: Pantheon.

Salzberger, Lotte. 1991. "Morbidity among Women from Disadvantaged Populations." In *Women's Health in Israel*, edited by Amy Avgar, 41–50. Jerusalem: Israel Women's Network, U.S./Israel Women-to-Women.

Sasson, Aliza, Charles Lewin, and Dina Roth. 1995. "Dieting Behavior and Eating Attitudes in Israeli Children." *International Journal of Eating Disorders* 17 (1): 67–72.

Sasson-Levy, Orna. Forthcoming. "Cross Dressing in the Israeli Military: Gender Identities among Women Soldiers in 'Masculine' Roles." In *Hear My Voice: Representations of Women in Israeli Culture*, edited by Yael Azmon. Jerusalem: Van Leer Institute and HaKibbutz HaMeuchad.

Scarry, Elaine. 1985. *The Body in Pain: The Making and Unmaking of the World*. New York: Oxford University Press.

Scheley-Newman, Esther. 1995. "Sweeter than Honey: The Female Discourse of Reproduction." *Text and Performance Quarterly* 15 (3): 175–188.

Schussheim, Eli. n.d. *In Anticipation of a Happy Marriage*. Jerusalem: Efrat Organization.

Scott, Judith A. 1984. "Keeping Women in Their Place: Exclusionary Policies and Reproduction." In *Double Exposure: Women's Health Hazards on the Job and at Home*, edited by Wendy Chavkin, 180–195. New York: Monthly Review Press.

Segal, Mady Wechsler. 1982. "The Argument for Female Combatants." In *Female Soldiers—Combatants or Noncombatants?: Historical and Contemporary Perspectives*, edited by Nancy Loring Goldman, 267–290. Westport, Conn.: Greenwood Press.

Sered, Susan. 1992. *Women as Ritual Experts: The Religious Lives of Elderly Jewish Women in Jerusalem*. New York: Oxford University Press.

———. 1993. "Religious Rituals and Secular Rituals: Interpenetrating Models of Childbirth in a Modern, Israeli Context." *Sociology of Religion* 54 (1): 101–114.

———. 1997a. "Arbiters of Female Purity: Conversations with Israeli Ritual Bath Attendants." *Narrative Study of Lives* 5 :40–58.

———. 1997b. "Women and Religious Change in Israel: Rebellion or Revolution?" *Sociology of Religion* 58 (1): 1–24.

———. 1998. "A Tale of Three Rachels, Or, The Cultural Herstory of a Symbol." *Nashim* 1 (1): 5–41.

———. 1999a. *Women of the Sacred Groves: Divine Priestesses of Okinawa*. New York: Oxford University Press.

———. 1999b. "Talking about Mikveh Parties, Or, The Discourse of Status, Hierarchy, and Social Control." In *Women and Water*, edited by Rahel Wasserfall. Hanover, N.H.: University Press of New England.

——. Forthcoming. "Religiously Doing Gender: The Good Woman and the Bad Woman in Israeli Ritual Discourse." *Method and Theory in the Study of Religion.*

Sered, Susan, and Ephraim Tabory. 1999. "'You Are a Number Not a Human Being': Israeli Breast Cancer Patients' Experiences with the Medical Establishment." *Medical Anthropology Quarterly* 13 (3): 223–252.

Shalev, Carmel, and Boaz Lev. Unpublished manuscript. "IVF in Israel—A Case Study for Rationing."

Sharoni, Simona. 1994. "Homefront as Battlefield: Gender, Military Occupation and Violence against Women." In *Women and the Israeli Occupation: The Politics of Change*, edited by Tamar Mayer, 121–137. London: Routledge.

——. 1995. *Gender and the Israeli-Palestinian Conflict.* Syracuse, N.Y.: Syracuse University Press.

Shatenstein, Bryna, and Jeremy D. Kark. 1995. "Mortality in Two Jewish Populations—Montreal and Israel: Environmental Determinants of Differences." *International Journal of Epidemiology* 24 (4): 730–739.

Shemer, Sara. 1992. *An Intimate Report about Israeli Women.* Tel Aviv: Sifriat Ma'ariv.

Skinner, G. William. 1993. "Conjugal Power in Tokugawa Japanese Families: A Matter of Life or Death." In *Sex and Gender Hierarchies*, edited by Barbara Diane Miller, 236–270. Cambridge: Cambridge University Press.

Sobel, Zvi, and Benjamin Beit-Hallahmi, editors. 1991. *Tradition, Conflict, Innovation: Jewishness and Judaism in Contemporary Israel.* Albany: State University of New York Press.

Solomon, Alison. 1991. "Anything for a Baby: Reproductive Technology in Israel." In *Calling the Equality Bluff: Women in Israel*, edited by Barbara Swirski and Marilyn P. Safir, 102–107. New York: Pergamon Press.

Spallone, Pat. 1994. "Reproductive Health and Reproductive Technology." In *Women and Health: Feminist Perspectives*, edited by Sue Wilkinson and Celia Kitzinger, 49–64. London: Taylor and Francis.

Swanson, Naomi G., Chaya S. Piotrkowski, Gwendolyn Puryear Keita, and Ami B. Becker. 1997. "Occupational Stress and Women's Health." In *Health Care for Women: Psychological, Social, and Behavioral Influences*, edited by Sheryle J. Gallant, Gwendolyn Puryear Keita, and Renee Royak-Schaler, 147–159. Washington, D.C.: American Psychological Association.

Swirski, Barbara. 1991. "Jews Don't Batter Their Wives: Another Myth Bites the Dust." In *Calling the Equality Bluff: Women in Israel*, edited by Barbara Swirski and Marilyn P. Safir, 319–327. New York: Pergamon Press.

Swirski, Barbara, Hatim Kanaaneh, and Amy Avgar. 1998. *The Israel Equality Monitor.* Tel Aviv: Adva Center.

Topley, Marjorie. 1974. "Cosmic Antagonisms: A Mother-Child Syndrome." In *Religion and Ritual in Chinese Society*, edited by Arthur P. Wolf, 233–249. Stanford: Stanford University Press.

Turner, Bryan. 1987. *Medical Power and Social Knowledge.* London: Sage.

Tuten, Jeff M. 1982. "The Argument against Female Combatants." In *Female Soldiers—Combatants or Noncombatants?: Historical and Contemporary Perspectives*, edited by Nancy Loring Goldman, 237–266. Westport, Conn.: Greenwood Press.

Van Esterik, Penny. 1988. "The Insufficient Milk Syndrome: Biological Epidemic or Cultural Construction." In *Women and Health: Cross-Cultural Perspectives*, edited by Patricia Whelehan, 97–109. New York: Bergin and Garvey.

Waldron, Ingrid. 1991. "Effects of Labor Force Participation on Sex Differences in Mortality and Morbidity." In *Women, Work, and Health: Stress and Opportunities*, edited by Marianne Frankenhaeuser, Ulf Lundberg, and Margaret Chesney, 17–38. New York and London: Plenum Press.

Wasserfall, Rahel. 1990. "Bargaining for Gender Identity: Love, Sex, and Money in an Israeli Moshav." *Ethnology* 29: 327–340.

———. 1992. "Menstruation and Identity: The Meaning of Niddah for Moroccan Women Immigrants to Israel." In *People of the Body*, edited by Howard Eilberg-Schwartz, 309–327. Albany: State University of New York Press.

Wegner, Judith Romney. 1988. *Chattel or Person: The Status of Women in the Mishnah*. New York: Oxford University Press.

Weiss, Meira. 1991. *Conditional Love: Parental Relations toward Handicapped Children*. Tel Aviv: Sifriat Poalim.

Wilkinson, Sue, and Celia Kitzinger. 1994. "Towards a Feminist Approach to Breast Cancer." In *Women and Health: Feminist Perspectives*, edited by Sue Wilkinson and Celia Kitzinger, 124–140. London: Taylor and Francis.

Wortman, Camille, Monica Biernat, and Eric Lang. 1991. "Coping with Role Overload." In *Women, Work, and Health: Stress and Opportunities*, edited by Marianne Frankenhaeuser, Ulf Lundberg, and Margaret Chesney, 85–110. New York and London: Plenum Press.

Yanay, Niza, and Tamar Rapoport. 1997. "Ritual Impurity and Religious Discourse on Women and Nationalism." *Women's Studies International Forum* 20 (5/6): 651–663.

Yishai, Yael. 1993. "The Hidden Agenda: Abortion Politics in Israel." *Journal of Social Policy* 22 (2): 193–212.

———. 1997. *Between the Flag and the Banner*. Albany: State University of New York Press.

Yuval-Davis, Nira. 1985. "Front and Rear: The Sexual Division of Labor in the Israeli Army." *Feminist Studies* 11 (3): 649–675.

———. 1997. *Gender and Nation*. London: Sage.

Zalcberg, Sima, Ayelet Berg, Dan Yuval, and Michal Ivancovsky. 1999. *Giving Birth in Israel: Findings from a 1995 Survey of Maternity Patients with Comparisons to 1993*. Jerusalem: JDC-Brookdale Institute of Gerontology and Human Development.

Zenner, Walter. 1965. "Saints and Piecemeal Supernaturalism among the Jerusalem Sephardim." *Anthropological Quarterly* 38 (4): 201–217.

Zola, Irving Kenneth. 1993. "Self, Identity, and the Naming Question: Reflections on the Language of Disability." *Social Science and Medicine* 36 (2): 167–173.

Zones, Jane Sprague. 1997. "Beauty Myths and Realities and Their Impact on Women's Health." In *Women's Health: Complexities and Differences*, edited by Sheryl Burt Ruzek, Virginia L. Olesen, and Adele E. Clarke, 249–275. Columbus: Ohio State University Press.

Index

Abergil, Linor, 100–2, 127
abortion, 2, 8, 10, 17, 20, 24, 28–40, 44, 53, 74, 147, 158–59, 163–64, 173
Abuhatzeira, Aharon, 31–33, 58
abuse, 67, 81, 87, 92–93, 135, 176
advertisements, 10, 63, 66, 101, 106, 127–28, 132, 148, 161; advertising industry, 8, 142, 148
Aharonovitch, Esti, 96–97
Amir, Delila, 36, 37
anorexia, 1, 21, 132, 151–53, 156, 158
Arab(s), 23, 28, 33, 73, 99, 133, 136, 139, 141, 149–50, 155, 171, 178; men, 133, 136, 149–50, 155, 178; women, 19, 101–2, 127, 152, 182
Ashkenazi, 24–25, 32, 42, 52, 56, 59, 107, 116, 147, 162, 173, 180, 182
authority, 14–18, 24–26, 30, 35, 39, 42, 44, 46, 52–56, 58–60, 64, 66, 70, 73, 91–92, 103, 105, 111, 113, 115, 118–19, 125, 134, 140, 143, 147, 152, 155, 157, 160, 163–66, 168–69, 172–73, 182
autonomy, 16–17, 26, 31, 118, 126, 159

basic training, 76, 79, 88, 178
Ben Gurion, David, 22, 47, 62, 130
Beniziri, Shlomo, 39, 81, 142
Berkovitch, Nitza, 22, 23, 25
Berkovitch, Einat, 130
Bible, 4–5, 22–24, 33, 37, 39, 41, 47, 60–62, 70, 81, 86, 106, 113, 116–17, 142, 146, 157, 165, 170, 173, 175, 182
birth allowance, 25–26, 28
birth grant, 25–28, 43
breastfeeding, 9, 20, 42, 55, 63–67
brides, 9, 20, 47, 100, 107–10, 113–21, 142, 164, 180
bus, 96, 135, 143–45, 148–49, 153, 155

caesarian sections, 43, 46, 123, 173
cancer, 3, 4, 11, 109–15, 122, 158, 172, 175
childbirth, 8, 9, 12, 16, 22–34, 41–67, 80, 88, 101, 104, 106, 113, 120, 159–60, 164, 173, 175, 180
Cicurel, Inbal, 107, 110–11, 113–15, 162
citizenship, 7, 14, 19, 25, 28, 61, 68–70, 73–74, 95, 98, 115
combat, 5, 9, 71–74, 78–79, 81–88, 90, 92, 96, 100, 102, 151, 157
commanding officer, 74, 77
consumers, 6, 7, 17–19, 66, 97, 114, 121, 124–25, 129, 140, 152, 162, 169
consumerism, 124–26, 152
contraception, 17, 37, 62, 177

Dayan, Moshe, 70, 91–92

Dayan, Yael, 130, 137, 139, 168–69
demographic "problem," 6, 20, 23, 26, 28, 30, 33–34, 45, 171–72
Deutsch, Yvonne, 99, 166, 175
diet, 4, 11, 45, 132, 158, 182
divorce, 20, 47, 100, 107, 114–16, 150, 180
Doyal, Lesley, 15

eating disorders, 87, 151, 182
Efrat (organization), 22, 38, 39, 173
ethnicity, 4, 19, 30, 32, 34, 42, 48, 55, 61, 107, 119, 147

family, 3, 10, 12–13, 16, 18, 27–28, 31–34, 38–39, 53, 56, 100, 106, 108, 113–15, 119–21, 142, 149, 151, 157, 162, 169, 171, 176
fashion, 10, 117, 124, 126, 130, 139, 146–48, 160–62
feminism, 2, 21, 30, 125, 129–30, 156, 160, 165, 169–70
fertility, 1, 2, 8, 28, 38, 41–42, 52–63, 66, 111–15, 131, 151, 160

Galili, Nir, 94–95, 101–2
gatekeepers, 44, 120, 163–64, 169, 182
gender, 2, 4, 5–7, 10–14, 20–21, 29, 32, 44, 68, 72–77, 81, 87, 92, 103–4, 115–16, 125, 138–41, 144–45, 154–59, 167–71, 176, 178, 180
gendering, 2, 6–8, 16, 19, 21, 74, 76, 78, 156–57
Grossman, Haike, 29–30, 34
guns, 52, 75, 77–90, 98–99, 132
gynecologists, 30, 36, 43, 106, 109–10, 117

Holocaust, 14, 24, 33, 65, 69, 169
hospitals, 6, 8, 17, 26–27, 35, 42–46, 49, 52, 55–59, 64, 67, 131, 164, 173
husbands, 12–13, 17, 31–34, 37, 41, 48–50, 53, 57–58, 63, 67, 72, 74, 80, 98, 110, 113–16, 120, 122, 142, 147, 149–50, 157, 162, 164, 182

Ifrah, Anneke, 3–4, 62, 64, 151, 171–72, 175–76
illness (sickness), 1, 2, 4, 6–7, 10–12, 20, 29, 35, 46, 54–56, 61–62, 87–88, 92, 103, 105, 110–13, 147, 156–57, 163, 166–68, 170, 175
impurity, 11, 47, 104–6, 112, 180
infertility, 9–11, 20, 23, 28, 30, 38–39, 41, 47, 56–63, 67, 111, 131, 160, 175
insufficient milk syndrome, 64
Israel Defense Forces (IDF), 5, 7, 9–10, 15, 17–19, 38, 69–102, 118, 123, 136–38, 145, 151, 155, 157, 164–65, 167, 176–78
IVF, 62–63, 175
Izraeli, Dafna, 16, 68, 69, 71, 75, 81, 86

Japan, 1, 12, 13
Jerby, Iris, 73, 74
Jewish law (*halacha*), 8, 40, 47, 50, 107–10, 112, 116, 118, 121, 139, 164, 175, 182
Judaism, 8, 19, 106, 126, 138, 148, 154, 166, 171, 182

Karasek, Robert, 14, 152
Kaveh, Ayelet, 107–8, 110, 112–14
kibbutz, 5, 152, 154
Knesset, 6, 8, 15, 19–29, 31–35, 38–39, 71, 74–75, 81–82, 92, 118, 129–30, 132, 136–37, 139, 141–43, 147, 155, 159, 164, 167, 173, 180–81
Koss, Mary, 5, 103, 178

labor, 17, 27, 42–46, 52, 54, 58–60, 66, 110, 116, 123, 139, 170, 173–75
Levy-Schreiber, Edna, 69, 78–80, 89
Lincoln, Bruce, 73, 104–5

marriage, 12, 20, 35, 39, 114–17, 122, 142, 152, 180
maternity leave, 6, 28, 64–65, 167, 173
media, 6–7, 10, 19–20, 61, 71–72, 79–80, 123, 125–27, 130–31, 143, 145, 151, 160, 167
medical establishment, 6–7, 10, 19–20, 25, 34–35, 45–46, 61–62, 66, 103, 151, 157, 159, 181
medicalization, 10–11, 29, 35, 44, 46, 65, 103, 106, 154, 159, 169

midwives, 22, 26, 42–45, 52, 56, 58–60, 64, 66, 160, 163–64, 174–75, 182
mikveh, 9–11, 20, 47, 60, 104–21, 162–64, 180, 182
mikveh attendants, 6, 10, 44, 64, 106–7, 110–21, 162–64, 182
militarization, 5, 19–20, 68, 81, 87, 91, 96, 103, 165–67, 175
military, 5, 7, 9, 17–18, 20, 51, 62, 68, 70–99, 103, 137, 140–41, 151, 155, 157, 164–68, 176, 178
Miller, Alice, 82
Ministry of Education, 16, 133–35, 155
Ministry of Health, 65, 172
Ministry of Transportation, 123, 144
miscarriage, 2, 50–51, 53–54, 63, 173
Misgav Ladach Hospital, 42, 46, 52, 63, 173, 181
modesty, 7, 117, 121–27, 133, 137, 141–54, 160–62, 181–82
motherhood, 8, 19–22, 27, 61–62, 69, 74, 86, 112, 151, 165–70
mothers, 12–13, 17–18, 20, 22–28, 31–32, 38–39, 42–43, 45–47, 50, 57–58, 60, 63–67, 70–74, 77, 86–87, 97, 107, 113–14, 120–21, 128, 151, 163–69, 176, 180, 182
myth, 8, 12, 23–24, 28, 33–34, 47, 51, 61, 69, 71, 104, 106, 116–17, 126, 166, 168

Na'amat, 99, 170
natural childbirth, 41–42, 45–46, 51, 53, 56, 159
niddah, 11, 20, 104–20, 162–63
North Africa, 1, 108, 120

Parents Against Silence, 167, 182
physicians, 1, 3, 8, 10, 16–18, 20, 31–32, 35, 38, 42–46, 50–53, 56–60, 62, 64–66, 105, 109, 110–13, 154, 156, 159–60, 164, 167, 173, 175, 182
pilots, 75, 80–82, 84, 91, 178
power, 7–8, 12–18, 29, 34–35, 37, 44–45, 61, 69–70, 73–74, 77–78, 93, 105, 125, 132, 138, 152, 154, 157, 158, 160, 163–66, 168, 170, 172–73
prayers, 17, 40, 48, 51
pregnancy, 1, 6, 12, 16, 26, 29–38, 42–64, 67, 81–84, 86–87, 110, 112–13, 120, 128, 159, 173, 175–76, 180
purity, 7, 9, 15, 23, 69, 86, 103–4, 106–7, 109, 112–18, 121–22, 124–26, 128, 134, 139, 141, 149–50, 153, 158, 160, 162–63, 166, 169

Rabbi Ovadia Yosef, 147, 161
rabbis, 8, 10, 17–20, 31, 42, 48–51, 56–60, 74, 105, 107, 111, 115–16, 118–20, 138–39, 143, 145–50, 153–54, 159–61, 164–65, 180, 182
Rabin, Yitzhak, 66, 70–71, 85, 130
Rachel (Biblical Matriarch), 22, 23, 28, 41, 48, 57, 58, 61, 62, 71, 166, 170, 182
rape, 5, 7, 20–21, 29, 69, 83–90, 93–98, 100–3, 127, 135, 141, 151, 165, 169, 178; Ramat HaSharon (rape), 96–97, 101
religious establishment, 6–8, 17, 19, 116, 118, 121, 137–38, 140, 142, 162–63
resistance, 21, 38, 46, 55, 73–74, 92, 155–70
responsibility, 14–18, 30–31, 36, 44, 52–53, 64, 66, 70, 73, 85, 112, 115, 118–19, 144, 152, 155–56
Resslan, Rena, 101, 127
rituals, 8–9, 13, 42, 47, 50–52, 55, 57–58, 61, 104, 106, 108, 113–14, 116–18, 120–21, 154, 159, 162, 173, 175, 180
Rosenblum, Pnina, 20, 124–25, 128–32

Sasson-Levy, Orna, 76–77, 84, 91, 176, 178
Schussheim, Dr. Eli, 39
scrutiny of women, 10, 20–21, 34–37, 75, 79, 116, 118, 120–21, 124–26, 135, 140, 146–47, 149–50, 153–54
self-defense, 5, 88–89, 178
sexual harassment, 5, 88, 90–93
sexuality, 7, 16, 37, 47, 69, 78–81, 86–87, 92–94, 106, 110–17, 120, 124, 131, 141, 148, 158–60, 162–63, 171
Shakdiel, Leah, 43, 172–76
Shas (Sephardi Torah Guardians Party), 33, 39, 81, 142, 147
sh'lom bayit (conjugal harmony), 33, 100, 113

Shostack, Eliezer, 23–24, 27
soldiers, 5, 9, 14, 51–52, 68–95, 103, 113–14, 126, 136–37, 151, 154, 164, 166, 169, 176–78. *See also* women soldiers

Torah, 24, 27, 33, 39, 49, 60, 77, 78, 138, 139, 140, 142, 149, 152, 157
Tsabari, Shoshana, 98

uniforms, 77–79
United States, 3, 4, 11, 34, 36–37, 39, 42–46, 53, 55, 60, 83, 90, 92, 99, 126–27, 138, 150, 171, 173, 175, 180

victims, 89–101, 134–35, 156, 159, 178
Vilenska, Esther, 6, 26
violence, 5, 20–21, 68, 81, 85, 87–88, 91, 93, 96–103, 128, 135, 140, 148, 157, 176
vulnerability, 5–7, 13, 46, 50–52, 61, 69–70, 73, 83, 86–89, 92, 97, 103, 105–6, 110, 114–15, 118, 146, 150, 162, 178

war, 23–24, 68, 71, 83, 85, 99, 137, 176, 178
Wasserfall, Rahel, 106, 115, 162
weddings, 47, 116–21, 140, 142, 160
Weizman, Ezer, 70, 80, 82, 130, 136, 178, 181
wigs, 146–47, 153, 161–62, 182
Women for the Sanctity of Life, 165–66
Women in Black, 137, 140–41
Women of the Wall, 125, 136–41, 157, 181
women soldiers, 5, 70, 73–74, 78–79, 80, 83–94, 101, 136–37, 151, 178
"womenandchildren," 7, 19, 74, 85, 99, 102–3, 136
Women's Army Corps, 70, 75, 78, 84, 92, 163–64

Yishai, Yael, 36, 98, 159
Yuval-Davis, Nira, 7, 69, 74, 84–85, 163–64, 175, 178

Zionism, 5, 12, 126, 152, 178